The HEALING POWER *of* Movement

DAVID & CHARLES

www.davidandcharles.com

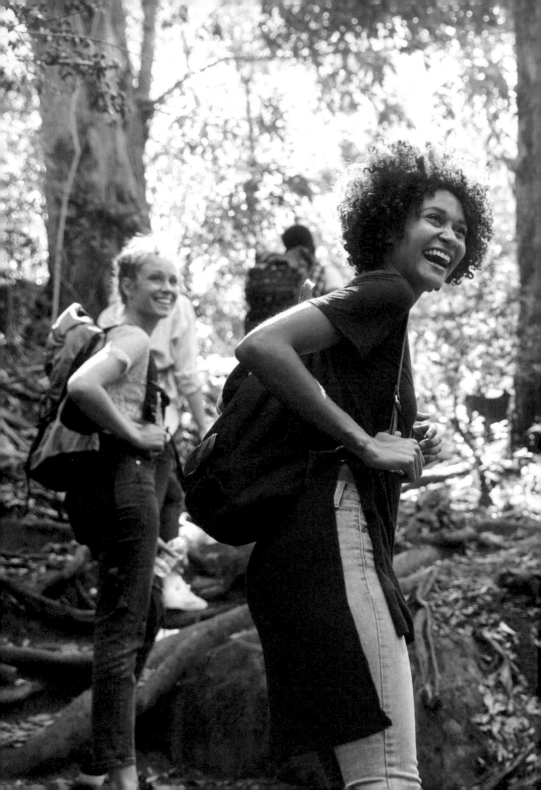

Contents

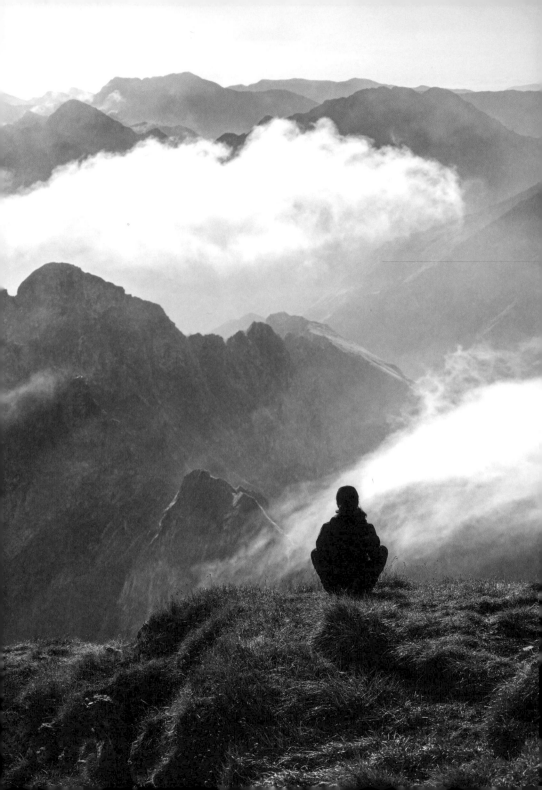

INTRODUCTION
Hello and Welcome

"The only way to make sense out of change is to plunge into it, move with it, and join the dance." Alan Watts, writer, speaker and philosopher

Welcome to being inspired to move with confidence and more freely. Welcome to letting go of the fear that you may not be good enough and might not be an elite athlete. Welcome to a tribe of amateur runners, walkers, yogis, and swimmers who seek health and wellbeing. Welcome to a place where exercise matters purely for the joy and enhancement it brings to our lives. In these pages, you will find words of encouragement, advice, and motivation to help you on your way into a journey of movement.

Ironically, fitness was never really my passion. In fact, at school, it was something I actively avoided. I'd go on an occasional run with my mum. Still, aside from being tolerable at netball, I failed in all conventional British school sports: tennis, hockey, football, athletics, and even rounders. I'd be the slightly lanky, gawky, glasses-wearing giant looming towards the back, avoiding the inevitable puffing of an often-inert non-athlete. I never loved exercise or the outdoors until much later in life.

It's funny now looking at how physical movement takes up such a large area of focus for me, how my ideas around training have developed and changed, how I've become accepting of my challenges to movement, and how I've begun to define what brings me joy. Walking, for instance, was something my parents filmed me screaming through as a child, stamping my feet, and crying. Yet somehow, I trekked multiple times through Nepal and the Lake District, so much so that I consider myself a part-time mountain goat.

Multiple reasons have led me to a more active lifestyle. Location is one of them. When mountains surround you, they become your home; lakes become your pools, and fields become your often-trodden path. Friends and family are also crucial; being involved by those who teach us techniques enables us to increase our confidence in new activities we may have otherwise never tried. My biggest reason, though, was a diagnosis of MS (multiple sclerosis) at 23, a condition that quite literally fatigues you and slowly degrades the quality of your immune system, balance, stability, and strength. Getting that diagnosis spurred me to try more, become a yoga teacher, trek to great altitudes and live as fully as possible. However, it also filled me with an apprehension that if I didn't start moving more I'd 'lose it', lose my ability to have the chance to try these things. I didn't realise it then, but movement in any way, shape, or form is one of life's most energy-giving and soul-sustaining aspects and led me to a healing path I'd never willingly have stepped on.

Movement, for me, has looked like many things. Some days it is simply increasing steps. Some days it is hiking up a hill. Some days it's drumming enthusiastically and vigorously in a samba band. There's no right or wrong way to move – there is only the time, space, and focus we give it.

When I think about my journey through movement, it has taken many forms. Every part of that journey has been for different reasons, but every portion has been reinvigorating physically, mentally, and spiritually. Movement has challenged me and forced me to reconsider ideas, to become more at peace, and to enjoy the moment. Learning to enjoy your body – its strengths and its stumbling blocks – has a profound effect not found anywhere else, and an effect I hope to help you recreate through this book.

A note on the text

In writing this book I realised there seems to be a natural link with an almost 'yogic' progression. First, we move the body, then control the breath, leading us to evaluate the mind better. For that reason, the book is divided into three main parts. Each will help you discover different aspects of what I now deem to be movement and hopefully inspire you to access new and different areas of your practice.

Feel free to work through the book linearly or play pick and mix, and indulge your freest and most curious spirit. Each section is written to give you the space to choose your path, your progression, and your practice, as it were. To help guide you on your way, on the following pages I've briefly outlined the types of information and advice that you will find in each section, including the activities and practices that are available for you to enjoy at your leisure.

MOVE WITH YOUR BODY

This section is about getting started and re-finding your simplest joy in movement. A practical guide to exploring different moving methods, whether swimming, running, yoga or walking. Initially, this section will guide you through a series of reflections to rediscover your 'joy' before moving on to starting practices in both yoga and running. After you begin your journey, you will focus on nurturing your body so that you may benefit most from your daily movement. Finally, the section will end with a breakdown of how to progress your activities further – take the plunge, as it were, into deeper practices and how to re-frame movement as a lifelong process.

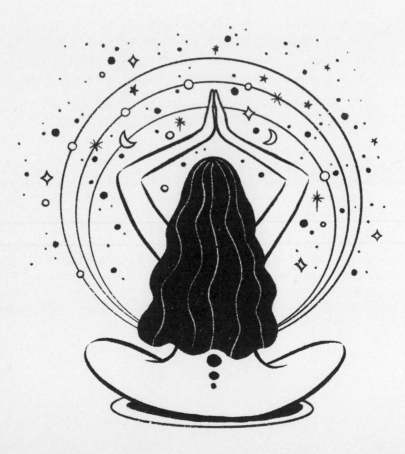

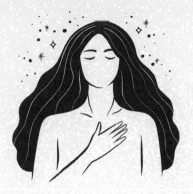

MOVE WITH YOUR BREATH

A huge part of the philosophy behind yoga is mastering your breath to regulate your natural emotional responses. There are many ways that these practices can enhance your movement and your general wellbeing and state of mind. We will be delving in this section into some of the science behind breathing and simple at-home practices you can begin to incorporate into your day. Again, this chapter will contain specific techniques for you to dip into as and when you wish but will hopefully serve as a resource for you to return to again and again to deepen your knowledge and confidence in working with your breathing.

MOVE WITH YOUR MIND

Finally, our last chapter is a reminder that resilience is built gradually. This section is a space for you to explore the fluctuations that prevent us from maintaining a consistent movement practice, and how to let go of any negative self-limiting thoughts that might hinder our moving process. With meditations, mantras, and mindful practices – this toolbox is set to equip you with a delightful array of methods to return to time and time again.

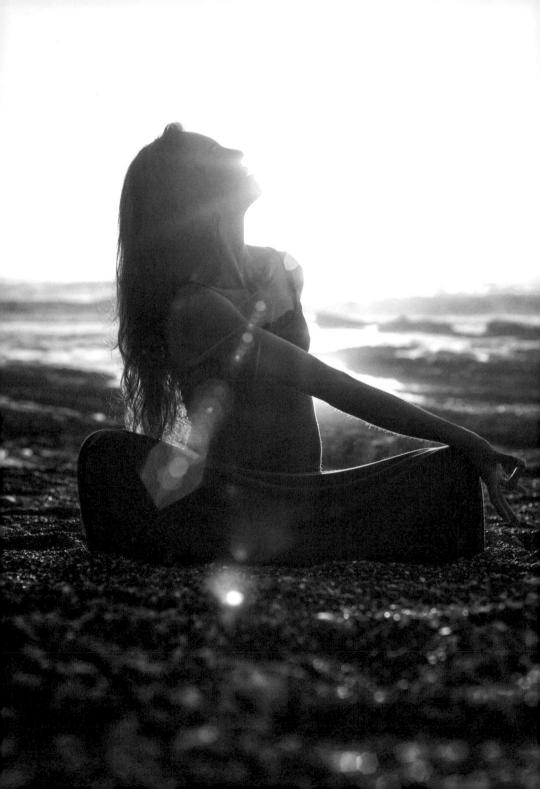

CHAPTER 1
Move with Your Body

"Movement is the song of the body."

Vanda Scaravelli, yoga teacher and author

In our fast-paced world, filled with endless responsibilities and commitments, paying attention to the power of movement isn't easy. We often find ourselves trapped in sedentary lifestyles, unaware of the profound impact that movement can have on our wellbeing. However, when we embrace the joy of movement we unlock a transformative experience that can heal our bodies, minds and souls.

To centre our focus on movement we first need to consider what we define as movement. Is exercise something that can only be done in a gym? Do you have to have the right equipment or clothes? Is it something we must turn up to even if we really don't enjoy it? The answer to all these questions is no. Movement is whatever we make it, whatever we find pleasure in doing. It can be something as simple as increasing our steps, beginning to jog or maybe even starting our own small yoga practice. Understanding the way in which movement has a fundamental effect on all aspects of our wellbeing can help us to reframe it in our minds – especially if we don't torture ourselves with an exercise regime that doesn't suit us.

This chapter is designed to help you move forward with understanding what movement means to you, and ultimately to help you navigate your own joy in movement.

Finding Your Joy

When we think about embracing movement, often it is with an unrealistic target of engaging in extreme lifestyle changes, which often don't bring us either joy or enable us to create sustainable movement routines. To establish good habits, we must first check in as honestly as possible with what we already do.

Mini check-in

Use these mini check-in questions as a baseline picture of your recent movement habits, or as a daily resource to help you keep on track. You could use the questions to prompt a reflection at the end of each day.

› How often did I engage in physical activity or movement throughout the day? Did I incorporate exercise into my daily routine, such as taking stretch breaks or walking?

› What types of movement did I engage in? Did I focus on structured exercises, such as going to the gym or attending fitness classes, or did I also include activities like walking, dancing, or playing sports?

› How sedentary was my lifestyle during the day? Did I spend prolonged periods sitting or being inactive? How can I incorporate more movement or breaks into my daily routine to reduce sedentary behaviour?

› Did I track or monitor my daily steps or activity levels? If so, what were the results? Did I meet my movement goals or targets? How can I adjust my routines to ensure I am consistently active?

› How did I feel physically and mentally after movement or exercise? Did I experience increased energy levels, improved mood, or reduced stress? How can I leverage these positive outcomes to motivate myself to move more consistently?

By reflecting on your daily movement habits, you can gain awareness of your activity levels, identify areas for improvement, and develop strategies to incorporate more movement into your lifestyle. Remember that every little movement counts; finding enjoyable ways to stay active can contribute to your overall health and wellbeing.

So, once we've reflected on our daily habits, what then? Successful incorporation of movement relies on understanding why we are doing what we are doing, how it impacts the body beyond increasing fitness levels, and then considering which approaches can be built into our lives over time.

The Physical Healing Power of Movement

Our bodies are designed to move. Movement is not merely a means of exercise but an innate expression of vitality. When we engage in physical activities, our bodies release endorphins, dopamine, and other neurotransmitters that elevate our mood and create a sense of joy. Regular movement improves cardiovascular health, strengthens muscles and bones, and enhances overall physical wellbeing. The healing power of movement manifests in increased energy levels, improved sleep patterns, and a more balanced immune system. Before redefining our movement through what brings us joy, we must first understand how movement connects with the brain.

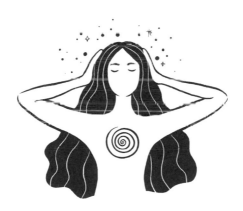

NEUROTRANSMITTERS AND MOVEMENT

Neurotransmitters play a vital role in facilitating communication between neurons in the brain and have significant implications for movement. Several neurotransmitters, including dopamine, serotonin, and acetylcholine, regulate and coordinate movement.

Dopamine release is crucial in connecting movement and our brain's reward system. When we engage in physical activity or exercise, dopamine is released in the brain. This dopamine release creates a sense of joy and satisfaction, motivating us to continue moving and exercising regularly. The anticipation and experience of movement-related rewards, such as achieving fitness goals, experiencing a runner's high, or simply feeling accomplished after a workout, can further reinforce dopamine release. This positive feedback loop between movement and dopamine release encourages us to stay physically active. It contributes to the wellbeing and overall mental health associated with regular exercise. Furthermore, it helps to control and coordinate motor functions by transmitting signals between neurons in the brain's motor pathways. Dopamine is essential in movement planning and execution. By understanding the link between dopamine release and movement, we can harness this natural reward system to help us maintain a consistent and enjoyable exercise routine.

Serotonin, another important neurotransmitter, regulates mood, appetite and sleep. It also plays a role in movement coordination. Adequate serotonin levels are necessary for smooth and precise motor control. Imbalances in serotonin levels have been associated with movement disorders such as restless legs syndrome and certain tremors.

Finally, acetylcholine is a neurotransmitter that plays a crucial role in the neuromuscular junction, where nerves communicate with muscles. It enables the transmission of signals from motor neurons to skeletal muscles, allowing for voluntary movement. Reduced levels of acetylcholine can contribute to muscle weakness and impair motor function.

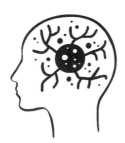

ENDORPHINS

Endorphins and movement are similarly intertwined, contributing to the positive and uplifting feelings often associated with physical activity. Endorphins are chemicals the body produces that function as natural painkillers and mood boosters. When we engage in movement or exercise, our bodies release endorphins, leading to euphoria and increased wellbeing. This release of endorphins can help reduce stress, alleviate pain, and improve our overall mood. It's commonly called the 'runner's high', which is the exhilaration and contentment that occurs during or after intense aerobic exercise. Regular movement and exercise can promote the stable release of endorphins, providing a natural way to manage stress, enhance mood, and improve mental and emotional wellbeing. So, by incorporating movement into our daily lives, we can tap into the benefits of endorphins and experience the positive impact they have on our overall happiness and quality of life.

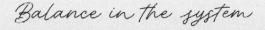

Balance in the system

> Overall, the intricate interplay of various neurotransmitters and hormones, including dopamine, serotonin, and acetylcholine, is essential for the regulation and execution of movement.

> Imbalances or dysfunctions in these neurotransmitter systems can have significant implications for motor control and may contribute to developing movement disorders.

> Understanding the role of neurotransmitters in movement helps shed light on the complex mechanisms underlying our ability to move.

The Mental and Emotional Healing Power of Movement

Beyond its physical benefits, movement has an extraordinary impact on our mental and emotional wellbeing. Engaging in physical activities allows us to disconnect from the demands of our daily lives and be present now. Whether dancing, hiking, swimming or practising yoga, movement serves as an avenue for self-expression, promoting mental clarity and reducing stress. Through training, we can release pent-up emotions, free ourselves from negative thoughts, and cultivate inner peace.

Movement plays a significant role in enhancing mental resilience and can positively impact mental stability.

Firstly, movement acts to reduce stress. As mentioned above, engaging in physical activity helps reduce stress levels by releasing endorphins, those natural mood-boosting chemicals in the brain. Regular movement can alleviate symptoms of anxiety and depression, improve emotional wellbeing, and enhance the body's ability to cope with stressors.

Secondly, as we have just learnt, movement is the great regulator of our moods and emotion. Remember, movement promotes the release of neurotransmitters like serotonin, dopamine, and acetylcholine, which regulate and balance our hormones. Regular physical activity can elevate mood, increase happiness and overall wellbeing, and provide a sense of accomplishment, improving mental flexibility.

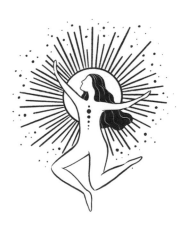

Movement increases cognitive function. Activity and exercise have been linked to enhanced memory, attention, and critical thinking skills. Regular physical activity boosts brain health, increases mental clarity, and improves your ability to adapt to challenges, strengthening mental resilience.

Building confidence and self-efficacy is another way that increasing movement can be viewed as a healing element in our lives. Setting and achieving fitness goals through movement can build trust and foster a sense of self-efficacy. Overcoming physical challenges and witnessing personal progress can transfer to other areas of life, helping us to develop resilience in various mental and emotional difficulties.

Similarly, movement increases mind-body connection and awareness. Movement practices like yoga, tai chi, and qigong emphasise the mind-body connection. By incorporating mindful movement, we can cultivate awareness, reduce stress, improve emotional regulation, and enhance our ability to bounce back from setbacks.

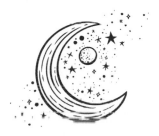

Finally, another recuperative benefit of movement is improved sleep quality. Regular physical activity can positively impact sleep patterns and enhance sleep quality. Sufficient and restorative sleep is essential for mental wellbeing and resilience. By promoting better sleep, movement contributes to improved cognitive function, emotional stability, and overall mental strength.

Incorporating regular movement into your lifestyle can have profound effects on mental resilience. Whether through structured exercise, sports, yoga, or any physical activity you enjoy, finding ways to move your body regularly contributes to enhanced mental wellbeing, improved coping skills, and the ability to navigate life's challenges with greater resilience.

Movement and Self-discovery

The movements we choose to make extend beyond the physical and mental realms; they are potent tools for spiritual growth and self discovery. When we move our bodies with intention and mindfulness, we tap into a deeper connection with ourselves and the universe. For instance, ancient practices such as tai chi and qigong blend movement with breath, harmonising our inner energy and promoting unity with the present. We awaken our spiritual essence through action, align our power, and open ourselves to a wider perception of ourselves and the world around us. This is where we truly begin to recognise our joy in simply engaging with our bodies physically and playfully.

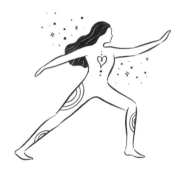

My first yoga class was simple; it was fitness based, intense and fast in an old school hall with about 20 other people. We flung ourselves up and down on our mats, and the sweat dripped heavily from my fingers. Until this moment, I hadn't fully enjoyed exercise, but I found with youth and flexibility that yoga made me feel strong. After a while, I became interested in what this practice was about. I went away, researched and realised that I might find a more mind-body-connected class that would progress my skills further. Delving deeper into the world of yoga, I engaged with mindful movement and breathing practices that filled me with a sense of collected calm and brought me joy – and still bring me joy to this day. I grew a love for the practice, and although it has developed and softened from my earlier days, there is a simple pleasure in returning to well-loved moves and holding that small portion of space for myself at the beginning or end of a day.

The joy of movement goes beyond momentary pleasure; it catalyses personal transformation. We confront our limitations and push beyond our comfort zones when we embark on a movement journey. We discover our resilience, inner strength, and ability to adapt. Movement challenges us to grow, to become more disciplined and focused, and to cultivate a positive mindset.

Now that we understand the healing power of movement, how can we cultivate it in our daily lives?

We begin by shifting our mindset and viewing movement as a source of joy rather than a chore. Find an activity that resonates with your interests and passions. This can be hard as there are so many choices. Experiment with different forms of movement until you discover what brings you the most joy and fulfilment, or consider using a guide to help you pick a few to start with.

I have often used the Ayurvedic (an ancient holistic healing system from India) method of 'doshas' (energetic bodies) to help me review which activities would suit my personality and body type. In a more Westernised world, we usually refer to particular body types as ectomorphic, mesomorphic and endomorphic to help define what exercises they would be most suited to; these tend to describe a person by physical traits only. However, the Ayurvedic system incorporates personality traits in the three types of dosha and prescribes movement based on a more holistic view of the person.

Vata, Pitta, and Kapha are the three doshas in Ayurveda. They represent the three fundamental energies or forces that govern the functioning of the mind and body. Each dosha has its unique qualities and characteristics, and they can be qualified in the following ways:

VATA

Vata is associated with air and ether (space) elements. It embodies qualities such as lightness, movement, creativity, and change. People with a dominant Vata dosha tend to have a slender body type and dry skin and may experience tendencies towards anxiety, restlessness, and irregular digestion when imbalanced.

PITTA

Pitta is associated with the elements of fire and water. It embodies qualities such as heat, transformation, ambition and intensity. People with a dominant Pitta dosha usually have a medium build, oily or combination skin and may exhibit tendencies towards perfectionism, irritability and digestive issues when imbalanced.

KAPHA

Kapha is associated with the elements of earth and water. It embodies qualities such as stability, groundedness, strength and nurturing. People with a dominant Kapha dosha typically have a heavier build, oily or smooth skin and may show tendencies towards lethargy, attachment and congestion when imbalanced.

According to Ayurveda, each person has a unique combination of these doshas, with one or two usually being more dominant. Understanding your dosha constitution can help you make lifestyle choices and adopt practices that promote balance and wellbeing. Ayurvedic recommendations include diet, exercise, daily routines and herbal remedies tailored to redress doshic imbalances. The following activity is a helpful guide to finding your balance of doshas; these will fluctuate at various points, so feel free to reassess whenever you think something has evolved or changed.

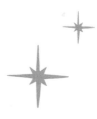

Mindful Movement

Ultimately, whatever you do, ensure you engage in movement
with mindfulness, allowing yourself to be fully present
in each moment. Embrace the challenges that movement
presents, knowing that they are growth opportunities. And
most importantly, find a community of like-minded people
who help you to get involved, enjoy and understand your
new movement practice.

ACTIVITY: FINDING YOUR DOSHA

For each question make a note of your initial answer, remember these can change over time so feel free to pop back to this quiz time and time again.

How would you describe your body frame?

a) Thin and slender

b) Moderate build

c) Larger and well-built

How is your skin texture?

a) Dry or rough

b) Sensitive or prone to redness

c) Smooth or oily

How would you describe your appetite?

a) Irregular or variable

b) Strong or intense

c) Slow or steady

How do you handle stress?

a) Feel anxious or worried

b) Get easily irritated or angry

c) Tend to withdraw or feel emotionally detached

What is your sleep pattern?

a) Light sleeper, difficulty falling asleep

b) Moderate sleeping, intense dreams

c) Deep sleeper, can sleep for long hours

How are your bowel movements?

a) Irregular or constipated

b) Loose or frequent

c) Regular or slow

How would you describe your body temperature?
a) Cold hands and feet, dislike cold weather

b) Warm body temperature, dislike hot weather

c) Generally tolerant of different temperatures

How is your hair texture?
a) Dry or frizzy

b) Fine or prone to early greying

c) Thick or oily

How is your digestion?
a) Variable, prone to gas or bloating

b) Strong appetite, prone to heartburn

c) Slow digestion, can skip meals

How is your mental agility?
a) Creative and imaginative

b) Sharp and focused

c) Steady and calm

What do your answers mean?
Calculate the number of responses for each dosha, and whichever is highest is your dominant dosha: a = Vata, b = Pitta, c = Kapha.

You may have a dual-dosha or tri-dosha constitution if you have an equal number of responses across two or more doshas. Remember, this questionnaire provides a general understanding of your dosha constitution. For a more accurate assessment, it's advisable to consult with an experienced Ayurvedic practitioner who can conduct a comprehensive evaluation based on multiple factors.

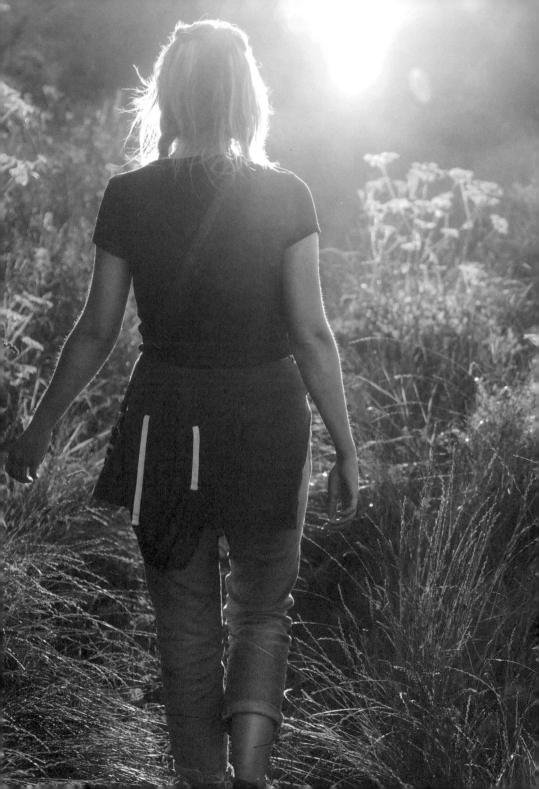

Nurture Yourself

So far, we have learnt why movement is good for our brains and bodies, but now we must discover how to nourish ourselves with movement.

Our propensity, particularly when we think of getting fitter or losing weight, is to jump to the extremes and believe that we can completely overhaul our lives in one go. We jump feet first into a diet or fitness fad, thinking it will cure all ills. Often this leads to unhappiness, sore bodies and starved bellies. You can probably see the recurring pattern if you've already made this leap a few times.

How do we avoid these negative patterns?

Simple, we make it sustainable, building new habits slowly, over time. We are trying to reimagine our often long-held habits and create space where we might otherwise see none.

BUILDING HABITS

Building habits takes time and comes with regular setbacks. It is a gradual process that requires consistency, determination, and an understanding of human behaviour. Whether adopting a new positive behaviour or breaking a negative one, you must gradually build up the pattern and reflect on how best to ensure it remains a constant habit. Reflection is key here. Reaching goals can often be perceived as a linear process. However, I like to view it as a winding path littered with spots for reflection and choices to be made. When we reflect, we consciously ask how and why something is or isn't working. We can assess where our choices were unrealistic and consider how to either alter aspects of a habit to be more sustainable or to let go of a habit that just isn't working for us.

Earlier, I asked you to consider what brings you joy, what you would really like to focus your movement goals on. It's easy to consider all the things we'd like to do and what might bring us that playful sense of freedom; the challenging bit now is to make them a sustainable habit and ensure that our activities can become meaningful parts of our existence.

Like any great foundation, we need something to work from, a realistic layout of our plans so we can retrace our steps if we lose our way and ensure the habits we start truly become sustainable. The following thought points and questions will hopefully help you create the foundations for this 'blueprint', ready to turn into a plan of action.

The Habit Blueprint

Here are some essential steps to build a habit effectively; with each step take a piece of paper and note down your initial responses to the ideas and questions proposed.

DEFINE CLEAR GOALS

› Begin by identifying the specific movement habit you want to build. Set clear and achievable goals to measure your progress. Make sure your goals are realistic and aligned with your values and priorities. For me past goals have been to combine music and movement – to drive down into something fundamentally rhythmic, or to increase my flexibility, or enjoy running in the fells around my hometown confidently. There is no one particular 'right' goal, and there is a world beyond simply getting fitter or losing weight.

Questions: Thinking about movement, what is your ultimate goal? To feel more energised? To increase flexibility? To feel stronger? Try to move beyond simple weight loss and consider the feeling of being able to move more freely. What will it bring to your life? How will you measure this? A diary? Your day in pixels?

START SMALL

› Begin with a small, manageable version of the habit. Starting too big can be overwhelming and demotivating. For example, if you want to start yoga, begin with an online or in-person class once a week rather than trying to practice daily. When I began to run in the fells, I set myself the target of a few smaller runs per week and one small fell run with a confident friend every other week. Similarly with cold water immersion, my goal was to go at least once a week to a local spot that was easy to walk in, with a confident group of outdoor swimmers.

Questions: How are you going to start, and when? If it's online, will you set aside a specific weekly time and build it into your schedule? Have you ensured that you have the right time for it, no other commitments are going to take precedent?

BE CONSISTENT

› Consistency is key to forming habits. Try to perform the activity at the same time or in the same context every day or every week. Consistency helps wire the habit into your brain's neural pathways. Like the earlier example of swimming or running, I have often found that every other day or once a week works best and then other events can be planned around that habit.

Questions: *How are you going to ensure consistency? What will keep you going week on week, day by day? Be honest. Write a mantra or motivational saying. Stick your schedule up in an obvious place.*

CREATE REMINDERS

› Set up reminders to prompt yourself to engage in the habit. Use tools like alarms, sticky notes, or digital apps to keep yourself on track. I find that scheduling a regular class acts as reminder enough, however when I decide to reach a goal without a defined class, I usually create events in my phone diary app for runs/walks etc in order to ensure I complete them. Another reminder I like to use is putting my clothes out ready; it's almost as if the clothes themselves talk me into doing the activity – especially an early morning run!

Questions: *What tools do you already own that will help remind you of your new habit routine? Do you use your phone for reminders or a bullet journal?*

BUILD A ROUTINE

> Incorporate the habit into an existing daily routine. For instance, if you want to walk more, then park further away from your destination.

> I frequently use this to readjust my habits – walking being a key one. I've found that if I keep headphones and an audio book handy, I can extend my dog walk and get some much-needed 'reading' done as well as increasing overall steps. Similarly, my other easy wins are parking further away from my work, making my bed the minute I get up so I feel more proactive, and giving myself until my second brew of the day to potter about before getting on with work or tasks.

Questions: What are your easy wins? Can you extend a dog walk or park further away from the place where you work?

STAY ACCOUNTABLE

> Accountability can be a powerful motivator. Share your habit-building journey with a friend or family member who can support and hold you accountable. Alternatively find small ways in which to hold yourself accountable. Personally, sharing goals with others has never helped me, however promising goals to myself has. A few years ago I really wanted to try and run a local fell race which took in around 4,000m (13,000ft) of ascent and 80km (50 miles) of landscape. I was nowhere near fit enough, however signing up to the race gave me accountability. I trained and gradually built up enough strength to run the race over some iconic fells. Accountability to me is about feeling a completion of personal challenge.

Questions: who are you accountable to? Can you list three people whom you can trust to help keep you accountable? Is there an event or goal you can sign up to in order to be accountable to yourself?

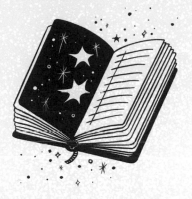

TRACK YOUR PROGRESS

› Keep a record of your habit-building journey. Use a journal or habit tracker to monitor your consistency and improvement over time. This could be daily or weekly. Or you could simply describe to a friend your recent smaller achievements such as running a farther distance, attending a class for an entire month or increasing your step count. No achievement is too small to track.

Questions: *How are you going to track your new habits? Are you going to keep a journal? Use an app? Talk to friends or family?*

POSITIVE REINFORCEMENT

› Reward yourself for sticking to the habit. Positive reinforcement strengthens the connection between the habit and the sense of satisfaction or joy it brings. The reward is usually the ability to maintain the habit itself, however it doesn't hurt to treat yourself to a nice yoga mat after a few months of solid practice, or to invest in a pair of awesome trail-running shoes after committing to a certain number of runs.

Questions: *What appeals to you as a reward? Can you link it to your new movement practice, e.g. a new swimming costume or tow-float for outdoor adventures? Try to build in definable rewards at certain points for consistency, not just for progress.*

EXPECT SETBACKS

› Recognise that building a habit is not always a smooth process. Expect setbacks and don't be too hard on yourself when they occur. Learn from them and use them as opportunities to adjust your approach. I like to see setbacks as opportunities for reflection – often I need to alter a habit, or even change to something else entirely if I encounter a setback. Some of the questions I like to ask at this point are:

Questions: *Does this habit really work for me right now? Have I simply achieved all I want from this current habit? Do I need to adjust the time, class, venue, activity, goal or reward?*

STAY PATIENT

Habits take time to form. Be patient with yourself and avoid getting discouraged if you don't see immediate results. Keep going, and eventually, the habit will become more natural and automatic.

› Once you have your blueprint, it's time to create your plan of action. Collate your notes into a workable plan. Stick your action plan somewhere visible – allow it to help remind you of what you want to achieve. Remember that building a habit is not about being perfect every day, but rather about making consistent progress over time. By following these steps and staying committed to your goals, you can successfully build positive habits that can enhance your life in various ways.

Nurture Your Body

Building habits is just one way in which we can ensure our movement is not only enhancing but nurturing our lives. In terms of nurturing our bodies, we can also look at how we practice movement and how we nourish our bodies with activity instead of draining them with the intensity of movement.

Take a moment and think about how you want to feel, say, after a run, swim, yoga class or other activity. What words come to mind? Energised, calm, exhilarated, supple, strong? Humans want to feel at our best: alive and engaged in our environment, not overworked, exhausted and adverse to the activity we wish to engage in.

At the start of this journey, we looked at how movement interacts with our brains and bodies and the benefits properly considered movement practices can bring. When I was teaching yoga full time, my biggest concern was giving space for students to progress their practice without overworking their bodies. Over the years, I noticed a few ways or 'tools' that seemed to help my students to move away from their over-competitive side and connect more with their intuitive selves. This intuitiveness is vital to creating a more nurturing environment for your movement habit.

One of my favourite practices for nurturing this more intuitive side of practice, is a mindful, subtle 'soft' yoga series called the Joint Opening Series. I wasn't taught to practice this way until I trained in Goa, India. However, it has been one of the biggest fundamental changes I have embraced in terms of becoming a more attentive movement practitioner. The idea is to stretch, flex and rotate from head to toe in a softly reflective and controlled way. You can do this using several movements, but I have suggested a simple routine to help you get started.

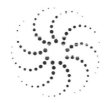

ACTIVITY: JOINT OPENING SERIES

EASY POSE

1   Find a comfortable spot on your mat or a soft surface. Sit with your legs crossed, bringing your left foot in front of your right foot and then your right foot in front of your left foot.

2   Rest your hands on your knees or thighs, palms facing down or up, whichever feels more natural to you. Allow your spine to lengthen, elongating through the crown of your head.

3   Gently close your eyes or soften your gaze, whichever feels comfortable for you. Bring your attention to your breath, taking slow, deep breaths in and out through your nose.

4   Feel the connection of your sit bones with the surface beneath you, grounding you to the earth. Allow your hips to relax and settle into a stable and balanced position.

5   Relax your shoulders, allowing them to soften and roll back slightly. Let any tension melt away from your face, jaw, and neck. Soften your forehead and release any furrows or creases.

6   Tune in to the sensations in your body, observing any areas of tightness or tension. As you exhale, consciously release any physical or mental stress, allowing your body to become more at ease and relaxed.

7   Maintain a gentle lift through your spine, finding a balance between being grounded and lifted. Imagine a string attached to the crown of your head, gently pulling you upwards, creating space in your spine.

8   Take this time to cultivate a sense of presence and stillness within yourself. Allow yourself to simply be present with your breath and the sensations in your body.

9   Remain in this Easy Pose for as long as feels comfortable to you, breathing deeply and calmly.

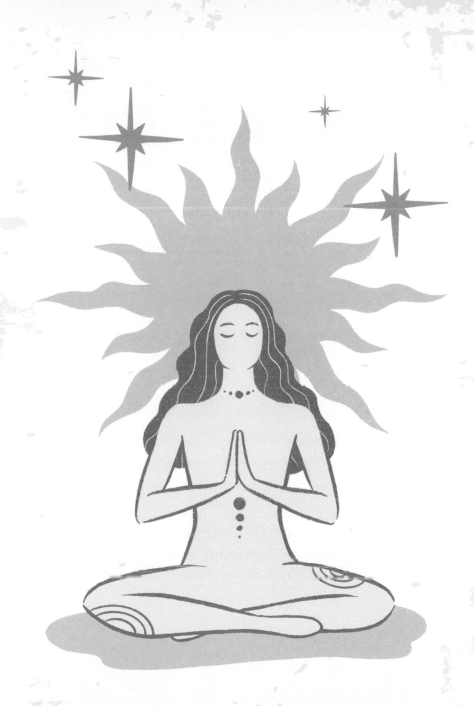

NECK SIDE STRETCH

1 Lengthen your spine and relax your shoulders.

2 Inhale deeply, and as you exhale, gently tilt your right ear towards your right shoulder, keeping your left shoulder relaxed.

3 Hold the stretch for a few breaths, feeling the gentle stretch along the left side of your neck. Feel free to intensify the stretch by gently placing the weight of your palm onto the side of the head. Be careful to add the weight slowly in order to avoid pulling too greatly on the neck.

4 Inhale and lift your head back to the centre.

5 Repeat the stretch on the other side, tilting your left ear towards your left shoulder.

6 Continue alternating sides, moving with your breath, and maintaining a relaxed and comfortable stretch.

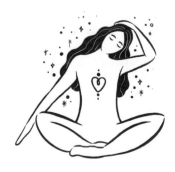

SEATED NECK ROLLS

1   On an inhale, gently tilt your head to the right, bringing your right ear towards your right shoulder. Allow your left shoulder to relax and avoid any force or strain.

2   As you exhale, slowly roll your head forward, bringing your chin towards your chest. Feel the stretch along the back of your neck.

3   On your next inhale, continue the circle by tilting your head to the left, bringing your left ear towards your left shoulder.

4   As you exhale, roll your head backwards, feeling a gentle stretch in the front of your neck. Be mindful not to strain or push too far.

5   Continue this circular motion, moving with your breath and maintaining a relaxed and fluid motion.

6   As you perform the neck rolls, be aware of any areas of tension or tightness. If you encounter any discomfort, adjust the range of motion or skip that direction.

7   Allow your breath to guide the movement, inhaling as you tilt or roll and exhaling as you complete the circle.

8   Perform several rotations in one direction and then switch to the other direction, ensuring balanced movement and stretch on both sides of your neck.

9   After completing the desired number of neck rolls, bring your head back to the centre and take a moment to notice the effects of the movement on your neck and upper body.

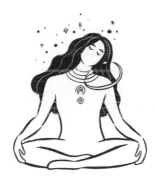

SEATED SHOULDER ROLLS

1 On an inhale, gently roll both your shoulders forward, bringing them up towards your ears.

2 As you exhale, roll your shoulders back and down, feeling a gentle opening across your chest and the back of your shoulders.

3 Continue this circular motion smoothly and fluidly, coordinating the movement with your breath.

4 With each roll, imagine releasing any tension or tightness you may be holding in your shoulders.

5 Pay attention to any areas of tension or discomfort, and if you encounter any discomfort, adjust the range of motion or skip the movement.

6 After several rotations in one direction, switch to the opposite direction, ensuring balanced movement and relaxation in both directions.

7 After completing the desired number of shoulder rolls, bring your shoulders back to a neutral position.

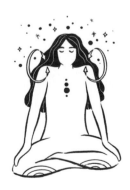

EASY POSE SIDE BEND

1 On an inhale, raise your right arm up towards the sky, lengthening through your fingertips.

2 As you exhale, gently lean to the left, bringing your right arm over your head and bending to the left side.

3 Keep your left sitting bone grounded, maintaining stability through your hips and pelvis.

4 Feel the stretch along the right side of your body, from your fingertips down to your hip.

5 Inhale, lengthening your spine and finding a little more space in your side body.

6 Exhale, allowing your breath to deepen the stretch as you gently deepen your side bend.

7 Be mindful of any sensations in your body, and if you feel any discomfort, ease off the stretch or adjust the position.

8 Hold the side bend for a few breaths, feeling the gentle opening and stretch in your side body.

9 On an inhale, slowly return to an upright position, bringing your right arm back down to your side.

10 Take a moment to observe the effects of the stretch in your body, noticing any changes in sensation or breath.

11 Repeat the side bend on the other side, raising your left arm up towards the sky and leaning gently to the right.

12 Return to an upright seated position to release the pose completely, finding balance and stability again.

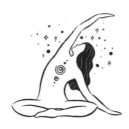

SEATED CAT/COW POSE

1 On an inhale, gently arch your back, moving into Cow Pose. Lift your chest, draw your shoulders back, and let your belly relax forward.

2 As you exhale, round your back, moving into Cat Pose. Drop your chin to your chest, draw your navel towards your spine, and round your upper back.

3 Continue this fluid motion, smoothly transitioning between Cat and Cow poses, coordinating the movement with your breath.

4 Inhale to transition into Cow Pose, allowing your belly to gently sink towards the floor and your gaze to lift slightly.

5 Exhale to transition into Cat Pose, pressing through your hands, rounding your back, and drawing your chin towards your chest.

6 Move with mindfulness and awareness, focusing on the sensation of your spine flexing and extending.

7 Find a rhythm that feels comfortable and natural for you, exploring the full range of motion in your spine.

8 Continue for several rounds, enjoying the freedom and mobility in your torso.

9 After completing the desired number of cycles, return to a neutral seated position, allowing your breath and body to settle.

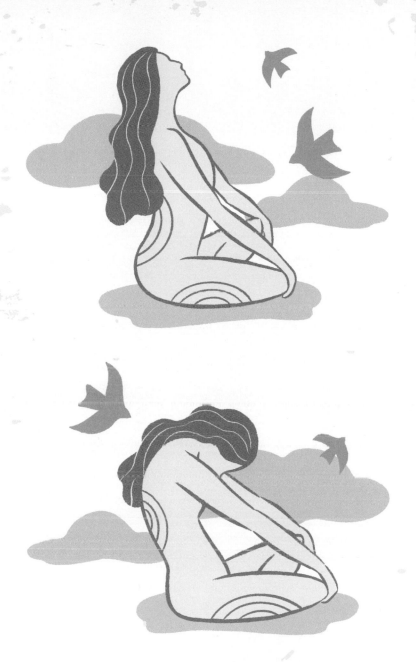

SEATED TORSO CIRCLES

1 Rest your hands on your thighs or place them behind your head for support.

2 Take a deep inhale, and as you exhale, engage your core by drawing your navel towards your spine.

3 Initiate the movement by gently rotating your torso to the right side, leading with your upper body.

4 As you continue the rotation, lean forward slightly and then circle to the left side, completing the circle.

5 Inhale as you reach the starting point, and exhale as you circle to the opposite side.

6 Maintain a fluid and controlled motion, feeling the gentle stretch and activation in your abdominal and oblique muscles.

7 Continue the circular motion, coordinating it with your breath. Inhale as you reach the starting point and exhale as you circle to the side.

8 Be mindful of keeping your spine long and avoiding any strain or excessive twisting.

9 If you encounter any discomfort or tension, reduce the range of motion or adjust the intensity to suit your body's needs.

10 After completing several circles in one direction, reverse the movement and circle in the opposite direction.

11 Be aware of any differences or sensations as you change direction.

12 After completing the desired number of circles, return to a neutral seated position with a tall spine.

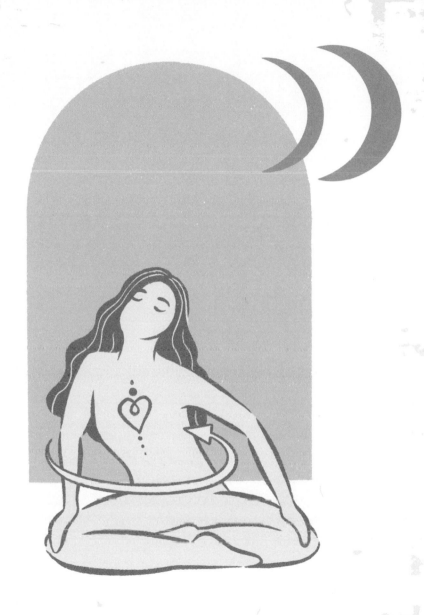

ARMS RAISED TWIST FLOW

1   Take a few deep breaths to centre yourself and bring your awareness to your body.

2   On an inhale, raise both arms overhead, reaching up towards the sky.

3   Lengthen through your fingertips and engage your core muscles.

4   As you exhale, twist your torso to the right, bringing your left hand to the outside of your right thigh and your right hand to the floor behind you.

5   Keep your spine tall and your shoulders relaxed as you twist, using your breath to deepen the rotation.

6   Inhale and lengthen your spine, finding more space in your torso.

7   Exhale and gently deepen the twist, allowing your breath to guide you deeper into the pose.

8   Stay in the twist for a few breaths, feeling the stretch along the sides of your body and the gentle rotation of your spine.

9   On an inhale, release the twist and raise your arms back overhead, returning to the centre.

10 Exhale and twist to the left, bringing your right hand to the outside of your left thigh and your left hand to the floor behind you.

11 Maintain a tall spine and relaxed shoulders as you deepen the twist, moving with your breath.

12 Inhale to lengthen your spine, creating space and openness.

13 Exhale to deepen the twist, exploring the full range of motion in your torso.

14 Stay in the twist for a few breaths, feeling the stretch and rotation on the opposite side of your body.

15 Repeat the sequence, flowing back and forth between the right and left twists, with each breath guiding your movement.

16 After completing several rounds, return to the centre and lower your arms, allowing your breath and body to settle.

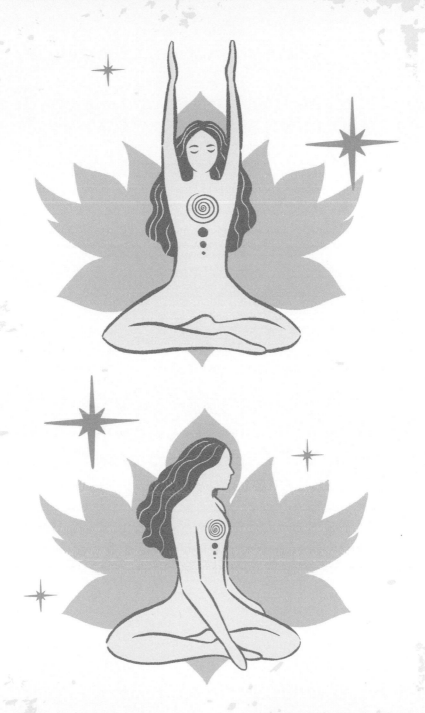

BADHA KONASANA INTO BUTTERFLY POSE

1. Bend your knees and bring the soles of your feet together, allowing your knees to fall open to the sides.

2. Gently hold onto your ankles or feet with your hands.

3. Sit up tall, lengthening your spine and keeping your shoulders relaxed.

4. Take a moment to find a comfortable position for your feet, adjusting the distance between them to a point where you feel a gentle stretch in your inner thighs.

5. If you find it challenging to keep your spine upright, you can place a folded blanket or cushion under your sitting bones to provide support.

6. Once you're settled, take a deep inhale, and as you exhale, allow your knees to gently lower towards the floor, working within your range of motion.

7. Maintain a relaxed and steady breath throughout the pose, finding a balance between effort and ease.

8. If it feels comfortable, you can gently press your elbows against your inner thighs to encourage a deeper opening in your hips.

9. Be mindful of any sensations or discomfort in your knees, and if needed, place additional support like blankets or blocks under your knees for added comfort.

10. Stay in the pose for several breaths or longer, allowing your body to relax and surrender into the stretch.

11. As you hold the pose, bring your attention to your breath and any sensations in your hips and inner thighs.

12. If you desire a deeper stretch, you can slowly fold forward from your hips to bring yourself into butterfly pose, maintaining a long spine as you reach your hands towards your feet or the floor in front of you. However, avoid forcing or straining in the forward fold and honour your body's limitations.

13. When you're ready to release the pose, use your hands to gently lift your knees back up and extend your legs forward.

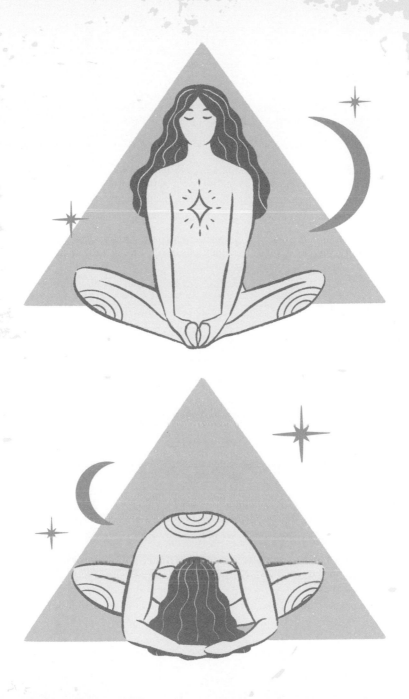

STAFF POSE INTO SEATED FORWARD BEND

1 Place your hands beside your hips, fingers pointing towards your feet, and press down through your palms to lift your chest and lengthen your spine.

2 Engage your core muscles by drawing your navel towards your spine, creating a stable and supported base.

3 Flex your feet, pointing your toes towards the ceiling, and press through your heels.

4 Ground your sitting bones firmly into the mat, maintaining a strong connection with the earth.

5 Relax your shoulders away from your ears, allowing your shoulder blades to slide down your back.

6 Imagine a string pulling the crown of your head towards the ceiling, elongating your spine and creating space between each vertebra.

7 Soften your facial muscles, jaw, and neck, finding a sense of ease and relaxation throughout your body.

8 Maintain a gentle, steady breath as you hold the pose.

9 Direct your gaze forward, keeping your neck aligned with your spine.

10 If you have tight hamstrings, you can slightly bend your knees to alleviate any strain in the back of your legs.

11 Use the support of your hands beside your hips to lift your chest and maintain an upright posture.

12 Feel the lengthening and activation in your entire back body, from your heels to the crown of your head.

13 Stay in Staff Pose for several breaths or as long as feels comfortable for you.

14 If you'd like to deepen the stretch, you can gently hinge forward from your hips, to bring yourself into Seated Forward Bend, maintaining the length in your spine as you reach your hands towards your feet or the floor in front of you. However, be mindful of not rounding your back or straining in the forward fold. Focus on maintaining proper alignment and listening to your body's needs.

15 Take a moment to notice the effects of the pose on your posture, spinal alignment, and sense of grounding.

16 To release the pose, gently come back to an upright position, using your hands to support your back if needed.

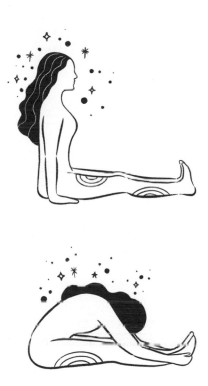

REVERSE TABLE-TOP POSE

1 Begin by sitting on your mat with your legs extended in front of you, your hands resting beside your hips, and your fingers pointing towards your feet.

2 Bend your knees and place your feet flat on the mat, hip-width apart, with your heels a comfortable distance away from your sitting bones.

3 Press down through your hands and lift your hips off the mat, coming into a Reverse Table-top position.

4 Keep your fingers pointing towards your feet and your wrists directly under your shoulders.

5 Engage your core muscles and press through your palms to lift your chest, creating length in your spine.

6 Gently drop your head back and allow your neck to relax.

7 Draw your shoulder blades towards each other, broadening across your collarbones.

8 Engage your leg muscles by pressing your feet into the mat, creating stability and support.

9 Be mindful of not sinking into your shoulders, and instead, actively lift your chest towards the sky.

10 Keep your gaze soft and forward, avoiding any strain in your neck.

11 Breathe deeply and evenly, allowing your breath to flow freely.

12 Maintain the pose for several breaths, feeling the opening and activation in your shoulders, chest, and hips.

13 If it feels comfortable, you can deepen the stretch by lifting one leg at a time, extending it straight out in front of you, parallel to the mat.

14 If you choose to lift one leg, maintain stability by engaging your core and pressing firmly through your supporting foot and hand.

15 Hold the pose for a few breaths, then gently lower the lifted leg back down and repeat on the other side if desired.

16 To release the pose, slowly lower your hips to the mat and extend your legs in front of you.

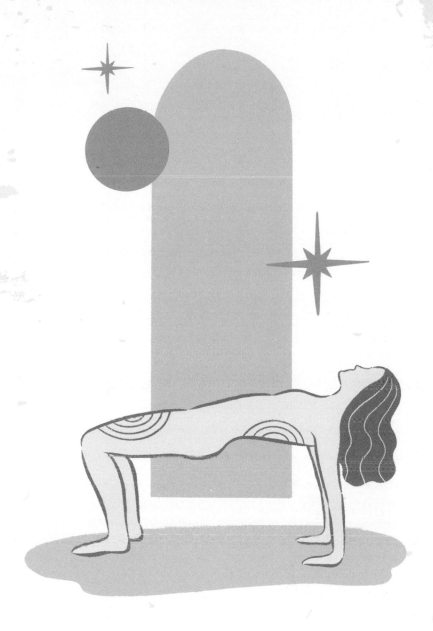

SEATED ANKLE ROTATIONS

1 Begin by sitting on your mat with your legs extended in front of you.

2 Bring your focus to your right foot and flex it, pointing your toes towards the ceiling.

3 Start rotating your right ankle in a circular motion, moving it clockwise.

4 Begin with small circles and gradually increase the size of the circles if it feels comfortable for you.

5 As you continue the rotations, maintain a relaxed and steady breath.

6 Feel the movement and stretch in your ankle joint and the muscles surrounding it.

7 After several clockwise rotations, reverse the direction and start rotating your right ankle counterclockwise.

8 Again, begin with small circles and gradually increase the size as feels appropriate.

9 Pay attention to any areas of tightness or tension and try to soften and release them as you rotate your ankle.

10 After completing the rotations in one direction, pause for a moment and notice the sensations in your right ankle.

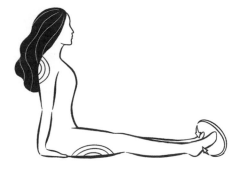

11 Repeat the same sequence of ankle rotations with your left foot, starting with clockwise rotations and then switching to counterclockwise rotations.

12 As you rotate your left ankle, bring your awareness to the movement and the stretch in your ankle joint and muscles.

13 Take your time and move at a pace that feels comfortable and safe for you.

14 Continue the ankle rotations for several rounds in each direction, allowing the movements to be fluid and smooth.

15 Maintain an upright and relaxed posture throughout the practice, keeping your spine long and your shoulders relaxed.

16 If you experience any discomfort or pain during the ankle rotations, reduce the range of motion or stop the movements altogether.

17 Remember that the purpose of this practice is to promote mobility and flexibility in your ankles, so be gentle and mindful of your body's limitations.

Enjoy the Joint Opening series weekly or if you wish, daily. Think of it as getting to know your body. There is no limit on how often you can do it, and taking it easily, gently and exploratorily will allow you to invest in yourself. Remember, this practice is about engaging with your mobility and flexibility with awareness. It is greeting your body with kindness and compassion and assessing your abilities safely.

Change Your Language, Change Your Mind

My natural personality is one of 'achieving personal bests' and 'can do' however over the years this had led to many injuries. I always told myself to push further, hold a pose longer, and found that in my yoga practice I was ultimately damaging joints and ligaments until I was forced to seek new ways to interact with my body and rebuild strength in overly flexible joints. On this journey, I stumbled across many interesting teachers and schools of thought who sparked a new perspective in my mind. This led to a more curious and open practice that supported my physical being instead of trying to conform it to an unnatural practice for my ability at the time.

It began with an introduction to the work of Peter Blackaby and his ideas on 'intelligent yoga'. His practice focusses very much on language and influence in practice. After workshopping with Peter, I realised that several of the cues I used created a forum for passivity instead of ownership. They commanded and did not invite. Now, this seems like a small insignificant thing to change, however language is incredibly powerful. Changing my language to be more invitational, with both my students and myself, opened incredible possibilities for movement. Instead of telling students to stay in place, I invited them to explore the posture, seeing where their comfortable limit lay and whether they could regulate their breath, muscles and strength within that space. Not only did this allow for students to push deeper it gave them the option to back away when needed; if the question was 'can you breathe a little slower?' and the answer was no, then a student would recognise that they needed to take a step back, resettle, restart with no fear or shame. Just curiosity.

Curiosity encourages exploration, creativity, and a sense of wonder in your movement practices. So how can we build this curiosity into our movement practice as a whole?

Well, through various strategies such as increasing awareness, changing up our routines as discussed earlier, varying long-held patterns, adjusting goals and challenges, reflecting and being open-minded to new possibilities.

REDEFINE WHAT YOU DO

Here are just some of the ways in which you could 'shake' things up and redefine your practice:

MINDFUL AWARENESS

By practicing mindful awareness, we focus less on the ultimate benefits of the movement and more on the present sensation of the movement at a moment in time – this allows us to be more adaptable to our body during the activity and less likely to cause ourselves harm. This is one of the key ways in which you can really shift your practices to be much more inviting and nurturing to your being. Begin by bringing mindful awareness to your body and movement. Pay attention to how your body feels, the sensations, and the range of motion as you move. Notice any areas of tension or restriction and explore ways to release and move more freely.

EXPLORE DIFFERENT ACTIVITIES

Don't limit yourself to just one type of movement. Try various activities such as yoga, dance, hiking, swimming, martial arts, or team sports. Each activity offers unique benefits and challenges, allowing you to discover what resonates with you. Look back at the section on Finding Your Joy and don't be afraid to let go of what is no longer purposeful or has ended.

EXPERIMENT WITH VARIATIONS

In your chosen activities, experiment with different variations and modifications. For example, in yoga, try different poses, props or flow sequences. In dancing, explore different styles and movements. Embrace the process of experimentation and let go of the need to perform perfectly. This can be applied to any form of movement and allows you to become a well-versed explorer in your continuing relationship with your own movement journey.

EMBRACE PLAYFULNESS

Approach movement with a playful attitude. Allow yourself to be curious, open to surprises, and willing to make mistakes. Playfulness can unlock creativity and encourage you to try new things without fear of judgment. In running, for instance, give yourself one run a week that involves quick bursts of delightful energy, run down a hill or incorporate skipping. In yoga you could experiment with silly or developmental poses that have a childlike nature in essence.

SET CHALLENGES AND GOALS

Challenge yourself to achieve specific movement goals, but make sure they are attainable and enjoyable. Celebrate each of your achievements and use them as steppingstones to keep expanding your movement horizons. Recap the section on habit building and techniques to keep yourself aligned.

MOVE IN NATURE

Take your movement practice outdoors. Nature offers a vast playground for movement exploration. Hike on different terrains, climb rocks, run on trails, or do yoga in a park. Being in nature can spark curiosity and bring a sense of wonder to your movement.

JOIN MOVEMENT COMMUNITIES

Connect with like-minded individuals who share a passion for movement. Join fitness classes, sports clubs, dance groups or online communities. Sharing experiences and learning from others can inspire your curiosity and keep you motivated.

IMITATE AND INNOVATE

Observe movement in others, whether it's a skilled athlete, a dancer, or a yogi. Imitation can lead to inspiration and new insights. Take what you see and make it your own, adding your unique flair and creativity to your practice.

PRACTICE MINDFUL MOVEMENT MEDITATIONS

Incorporate mindfulness and movement in meditative practices. Focus your attention on the sensations of each movement, breathing, and the present moment. This deepens your connection to your body and enhances your curiosity.

REFLECT AND JOURNAL

Keep a movement journal to document your experiences, insights, and discoveries. Reflect on how movement affects your mood, energy levels, and overall wellbeing. This self-awareness can help you refine your movement practice and embrace curiosity.

Let curiosity be your guide

› Remember that curiosity in movement is a continuous journey.

› Embrace the exploration process and be kind to yourself as you try new things.

› Stay open to surprises and find joy in the ever-evolving nature of movement.

› Let curiosity be your guide to a lifelong and fulfilling relationship with physical activity.

ACTIVITY: SPINAL RESET

Why not try out your new-found ideas on exploration and curiosity in a practice I love, the Spinal Reset? I consider this to be one of the most nurturing practices to come back to, particularly when you feel a need to simply breathe and reconnect.

CONSTRUCTIVE REST POSE OR SEMI-SAVASANA

1   Set up your space. Find a quiet and comfortable place where you can lie down. Use a yoga mat or a soft surface like a carpet or blanket to cushion your body.

2   Start by lying down on your back. Extend your legs straight out on the mat and let your feet fall naturally to the sides.

3   Gently bend your knees. Keep both your feet flat on the mat, feeling for an even footprint.

4   Allow your arms to rest comfortably alongside your body with your palms facing up. Keep your shoulders relaxed and away from your ears.

5   Softly close your eyes or gaze at a fixed point to turn your focus inward.

6   Take a moment to adjust your body, ensuring that you're comfortable and fully supported by the surface beneath you.

7   Take slow and deep breaths, inhaling through your nose and exhaling through your mouth. Let go of any tension or stress with each exhalation.

8   Remain in Constructive Rest with bent legs for 3 to 5 minutes. Allow your mind to quieten down and your body to relax completely.

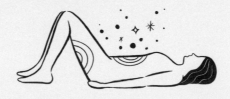

Alternative Hip Forward Flow Whilst in this position begin to gently lift alternate hips so that they hover only millimetres from the ground, you should feel the movement of your knees, moving forward and a tilting from side to side, in your hips.

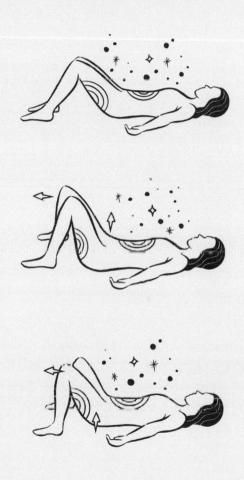

SUPINE SPINAL TWIST

1 Return to Constructive Rest and gently bend your knees bringing them toward your chest.

2 Inhale and as you exhale, drop both knees to the right side of your body. Keep your knees together if possible.

3 Extend your arms out to the sides, forming a 'T' shape with your body. Keep your shoulders grounded and relaxed.

4 Turn your head to the left, looking in the opposite direction to your knees.

5 Take deep breaths and try to relax your body into the twist. You should feel a gentle stretch along your spine and possibly in your hips.

6 Hold the Supine Spinal Twist for 30 seconds to 1 minute, or longer if it feels comfortable. Focus on breathing deeply and letting go of any tension in your body.

7 To come out of the pose, inhale and bring your knees back to the centre. Take a moment to neutralise your spine by extending your legs out straight. Then, repeat the twist on the other side by lowering your legs to the left and turning your head to the right.

8 After completing both sides, bring your knees back to the centre and hug them into your chest for a moment.

9 You can make the pose dynamic by moving with the breath from side to side. Inhale to centre, exhale to twist.

10 Release your legs and arms and stretch them out fully. Relax in Savasana (see the final pose in this Spinal Reset sequence) for a few breaths to allow your body to absorb the benefits of the twist.

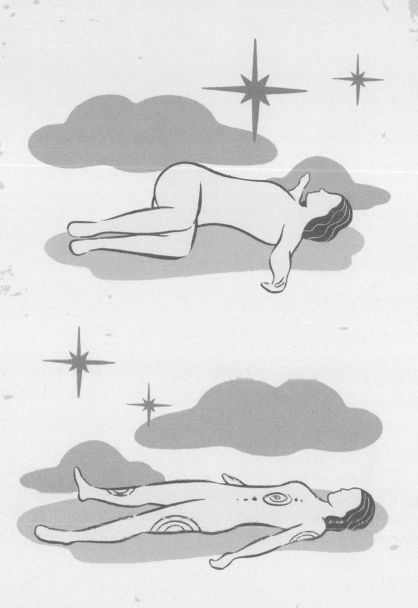

1 Next, find a neutral spine position. This means that your natural curves in the lower back (lumbar), middle back (thoracic), and neck (cervical) are all present and not exaggerated or flattened.

2 Inhale to prepare, and as you exhale, gently engage your abdominal muscles and tilt your pelvis backward, pressing your lower back into the mat. Imagine that you are trying to flatten your lower back against the floor.

3 Continue to engage your abdominal muscles as you tuck your tailbone slightly and lift your hips a few inches off the mat. Your feet should remain on the ground.

4 Hold the Supine Pelvic Tilt Tuck for a few seconds while maintaining the engagement in your core and the lift in your hips.

5 Inhale and slowly release the tilt and tuck, lowering your hips back down to the mat.

6 Perform 8 to 10 repetitions of the Supine Pelvic Tilt Tuck, focusing on the controlled movement and proper engagement of your core muscles.

Tips

Avoid arching your back excessively during this exercise. The movement should come from your pelvis and core muscles, not from your lower back.

Keep your breathing steady and controlled throughout the exercise. Exhale as you tilt and tuck, and inhale as you release.

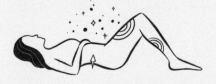 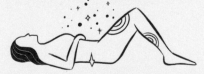

BRIDGE POSE

1 Lie with your knees bent and your feet flat on the floor, making sure your feet are hip-width apart and close to your sitting bones.

2 Let your arms rest alongside your body with your palms facing down. Your fingertips should be lightly touching your heels.

3 Take a deep breath in and as you exhale, press your feet firmly into the floor. Engage your glutes (buttock muscles) and core muscles.

4 Inhale and slowly begin to lift your hips off the mat, raising them towards the ceiling. Keep pressing through your feet and shoulders to lift your hips higher.

5 Roll your shoulders slightly underneath your body, and clasp your hands together if you can. This will help open your chest and create a stable base for the pose.

6 Make sure your neck and head are relaxed. You can keep your gaze straight up or gently tuck your chin to your chest.

7 As you hold the pose, continue to press through your feet and engage your glutes and core to keep your hips lifted and stable.

8 Take deep and even breaths while holding the pose for about 30 seconds to 1 minute, depending on your comfort level and strength.

9 To come out of Bridge Pose, gently unclasp your hands and slowly lower your hips back down to the mat one vertebra at a time.

10 Take a moment to rest in Savasana or Corpse Pose and observe the effects of the pose on your body. If desired, you can repeat Bridge Pose for another round.

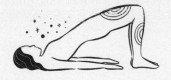

Give yourself the space to explore a more dynamic Bridge Pose by lifting your arms overhead and stretching them beyond the ears on the inhale, lowering and stretching the fingers towards the toes on the exhale.

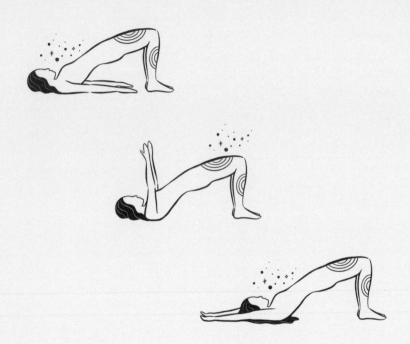

Tips

Avoid excessive arching in the lower back. Engage your core muscles to support your lower back and protect your spine.

Keep your knees hip-width apart and avoid letting them splay outward.

If clasping your hands is difficult, you can keep your arms alongside your body with palms facing down.

SUPINE TOE TAPS FLOW

1 Return to bent knees and place your feet flat on the floor, hip-width apart.

2 Take a deep breath in, and as you exhale, engage your core muscles by drawing your navel towards your spine. This will create stability in your lower back.

3 Keeping your knees bent, lift your feet off the floor, so your shins are parallel to the ground. Your thighs should be perpendicular to the ground, creating a 90-degree angle at your knees.

4 From this position, start to tap one foot down towards the floor while keeping your core engaged and your lower back flat on the mat. Only tap your toes lightly on the ground and avoid letting your lower back arch.

5 Lift the foot you tapped down and return it to the starting position. Then, lower the other foot to tap the toes on the floor. Continue to alternate legs in a controlled and coordinated manner.

6 Coordinate your breath with the movement. Exhale as you tap one foot down, and inhale as you bring it back up. Repeat the same breathing pattern for the other leg.

7 While performing the toe taps, keep your upper body relaxed and shoulders away from your ears.

8 Focus on maintaining stability in your core throughout the exercise. Avoid any rocking or swinging motions and keep the movement controlled.

9 Start with 10 to 15 repetitions per leg (20 to 30 taps in total). You can perform 2 to 3 sets depending on your fitness level and preference.

10 After completing the sets, lower your feet to the floor and rest for a moment, observing the effects of the exercise on your core muscles.

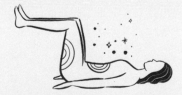 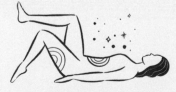

DEAD BUG CORE SERIES

1   Bend your knees and lift your feet off the floor, so your knees are directly above your hips. Your shins should be parallel to the floor, creating a 90-degree angle at your knees.

2   Extend your arms straight up toward the ceiling, perpendicular to the floor. Your palms should face each other, and your shoulders should be relaxed.

3   Take a deep breath in, and as you exhale, engage your core muscles by drawing your navel towards your spine. This will create stability in your lower back.

4   As you exhale, simultaneously extend your right arm overhead toward the floor behind you and straighten your left leg out, hovering it a few inches above the floor. Keep your lower back pressed into the mat throughout the movement.

5   Inhale as you bring your right arm and left leg back to the starting position, with your knees bent and your feet lifted off the floor.

6   Exhale again, this time extending your left arm overhead and straightening your right leg out. Keep your core engaged as you move.

7   Continue alternating sides, reaching one arm and the opposite leg away from your body while keeping your core stable. Perform the movement in a controlled and coordinated manner.

8   Coordinate your breath with the movement. Exhale as you extend your arm and leg, and inhale as you return to the starting position.

9   Focus on maintaining stability in your core throughout the exercise. Avoid arching your back or lifting your head and shoulders off the mat.

10 Start with 10 to 12 repetitions on each side (20 to 24 repetitions in total). You can perform 2 to 3 sets depending on your fitness level and preference.

11 After completing the sets, lower your feet to the floor, rest for a moment, and observe the effects of the exercise on your core muscles.

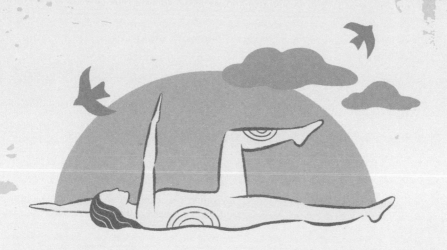

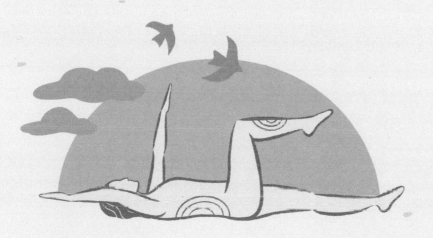

RECLINED KNEE CIRCLES

1 Keeping your core engaged, lift your right knee towards your chest, bringing it as close as comfortable. Hold your right knee with both hands to support the movement.

2 Start to make small circles with your right knee in a clockwise direction. The circles should be smooth and controlled, and the movement should originate from your hip joint.

3 After a few circles in one direction, reverse the movement, and make circles in a counterclockwise direction with your right knee.

4 After completing circles with your right knee, release your right leg back to the floor. Repeat the same movement with your left knee, making circles in both clockwise and counterclockwise directions.

5 Throughout the exercise, focus on keeping your lower back flat on the mat and your core engaged. Avoid arching your back or lifting your shoulders off the floor.

6 Coordinate your breath with the movement. Inhale as you start the circle, and exhale as you complete one full circle.

7 Aim to perform 6 to 10 circles in each direction with each leg.

8 After completing the circles with both legs, now feel free to circle both knees together in order to massage into the lower back. Release your legs back to the floor, rest for a moment, and observe the effects of the exercise on your hip joints and lower back.

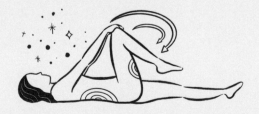

WIND RELEASE POSE FLOW

1   Now, from Constructive Rest or Semi-savasana Pose, bend both knees and bring them toward your chest as you exhale. Wrap your arms around your legs, hugging them gently. Your hands can hold the opposite elbows or you can clasp your fingers below your knees.

2   As you inhale, release the hug on your knees and extend your legs back out straight on the mat.

3   Repeat the movement by exhaling and bringing your knees back toward your chest, hugging them gently with your arms.

4   Coordinate your breath with the movement. Exhale as you hug your knees into your chest, and inhale as you release your legs away from the chest holding o to the knees.

5   Repeat the flow for 3 to 5 rounds (or more if you wish), maintaining a steady and smooth rhythm of exhaling and hugging your knees, followed by inhaling and releasing your legs.

6   After completing the flow rounds, release your knees and lie flat on your back. Take a few deep breaths in and out, allowing your body to relax and settle.

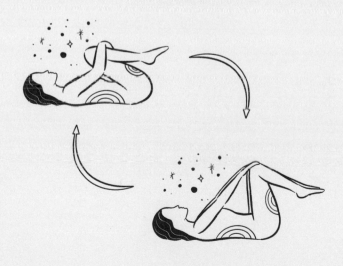

ROCKING AND ROLLING

1 On an exhale, bend your knees and bring them toward your chest. Wrap your arms around your knees, holding onto your shins or clasping your hands together below your knees.

2 Hug your knees gently, drawing them as close to your chest as feels comfortable. Keep your neck and shoulders relaxed throughout the movement.

3 Inhale deeply and as you exhale, start to rock backward, gently rolling onto your upper back and shoulders. Use the momentum to rock back up to the starting position.

4 Inhale as you rock forward, drawing your knees closer to your chest. Exhale as you rock backward, rolling onto your upper back and shoulders. Keep the movement fluid and rhythmic.

5 Engage your core muscles to control the rocking motion, and synchronise your breath with the movement. Inhale as you rock forward, and exhale as you rock backward.

6 If you have any neck or back issues, perform the rocking motion with smaller movements, keeping your head and shoulders gently on the ground.

7 After about 3 to 5 rounds of rocking, come to stillness in a hugging position with your knees drawn toward your chest.

8 Release your knees and extend your legs out straight on the mat. Take a moment to rest and observe the effects of the rocking motion on your body.

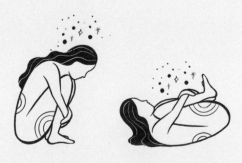

PLOUGH POSE

1 Lie down on your yoga mat with your legs extended and arms resting alongside your body, palms facing down.

2 Inhale deeply, and as you exhale, engage your core muscles. Lift your legs off the ground, and bring them overhead towards the floor behind you.

3 Place your hands on your lower back for support. Your palms should be on the upper part of your back, with your fingers pointing towards your hips.

4 Continue to use your core strength to lift your hips higher, bringing your toes as close to the ground as you comfortably can.

5 As you hold the pose, try to maintain a straight line from your glutes to your heels. Keep your neck relaxed and gaze straight up or towards your toes.

6 Take deep and steady breaths as you hold the pose. Keep your breathing smooth and avoid straining or holding your breath.

7 When you are ready to come out of the pose, use your hands for support as you slowly roll your spine back down to the mat, one vertebra at a time.

8 After releasing the pose, lie flat on your back in Savasana or Corpse Pose to allow your body to rest and recover.

Note Plough Pose is an intermediate to advanced yoga pose that requires flexibility and strength in the spine, shoulders, and hamstrings. Placing the hands on the back can provide extra support and make the pose more accessible. However, it's essential to proceed with caution and avoid any strain on the neck or lower back. If you are new to this pose or have any existing neck or back issues, it's recommended to practice under the guidance of an experienced yoga instructor. Avoid this pose if you have any recent injuries, high blood pressure, or other medical conditions that could be affected by inversions.

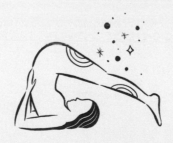

FISH POSE

1   Lie down on your yoga mat with your legs extended and your arms resting alongside your body, palms facing down. Take a moment to relax and find a comfortable position.

2   Slide your hands under your hips, with your palms facing down and your forearms pressing into the mat. This will provide support for your lower back during the back bend.

3   Inhale deeply, and as you exhale, press your forearms and elbows firmly into the mat, lifting your chest and head off the ground. Arch your upper back and gently tilt your head back, allowing the crown of your head to rest lightly on the floor.

4   Optional: For a deeper stretch, you can lift your heart higher by straightening your arms and pointing your fingers toward your feet. Keep pressing your elbows into the mat to support your lower back.

5   Draw your shoulder blades toward each other to open your chest even more. Keep your neck relaxed and avoid straining the muscles in your neck.

6   Take deep breaths and try to relax into the pose. Feel the expansion in your chest and front of the body with each inhale.

7   Stay in Fish Pose for 30 seconds to 1 minute, depending on your comfort level. If you feel any discomfort or strain, come out of the pose slowly.

8   To come out of the pose, tuck your chin into your chest and lower your chest and head back down to the mat. Slide your hands out from under your hips and rest them alongside your body.

9   After releasing the pose, lie flat on your back in Savasana or Corpse Pose to rest and integrate the benefits of the back bend.

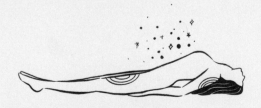

SUPINE WINDSHIELD WIPERS

1 Lie down on your yoga mat with your legs extended and your arms resting alongside your body, palms facing down, or spread out to the sides.

2 Inhale deeply, and as you exhale, bend your knees and draw them towards your chest.

3 Bring your knees together and then let them fall to one side of your body, towards the floor. Keep your shoulders and hips grounded on the mat.

4 Turn your head in the opposite direction to your knees. For example, if your knees are falling to the right, turn your head to the left.

5 Hold the Supine Windshield Wipers pose for a few breaths, feeling the stretch in your hips and lower back.

6 Inhale as you bring your knees back to the centre, hugging them into your chest.

7 Exhale and let your knees fall to the opposite side of your body, while turning your head to look in the opposite direction.

8 Repeat the windshield wiper motion by gently moving your knees from side to side, while keeping your shoulders and hips grounded on the mat.

9 Coordinate your breath with the movement. Inhale as you bring your knees back to the centre, and exhale as you let them fall to the side.

10 After about 3 to 5 rounds, release the pose by extending your legs back out straight on the mat.

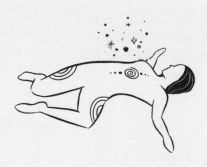

BANANA POSE

1. Lie down on your yoga mat with your legs extended and your arms resting alongside your body, palms facing down.

2. Keep your feet together and your legs straight.

3. Inhale deeply, and as you exhale, stretch your arms overhead, reaching them towards the opposite end of your mat. Lengthen your entire body from your fingers to your toes.

4. As you inhale, begin to arch your body to one side, creating a gentle crescent shape. Keep both shoulders and hips grounded on the mat.

5. You should feel a deep stretch along the entire side of your body on the side you are arching away from. This will target the ribs, waist, and hips.

6. Hold the pose for a few breaths, breathing deeply and allowing the stretch to deepen with each exhale.

7. Inhale and come back to the centre, stretching your arms overhead again.

8. Exhale and arch your body to the opposite side, creating the crescent shape on the other side of your body.

9. Stay in the Banana Pose on this side for a few breaths, enjoying the stretch along the opposite side of your body.

10. Inhale and return to the centre, stretching your arms overhead one more time.

11. Exhale and release your arms, relaxing them alongside your body. Take a moment to observe the effects of the stretch on both sides of your body.

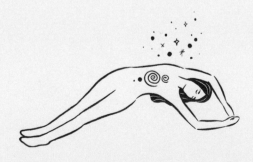

RECLINING BOUND ANGLE POSE

1. Lie down on your yoga mat with your legs extended and your arms resting alongside your body, palms facing down, or out from your sides depending on your preference.

2. Bend your knees and bring the soles of your feet together, allowing your knees to fall open to the sides. Your feet should be a comfortable distance away from your pelvis.

3. Slide your feet closer to or farther away from your body, depending on your flexibility. The closer your feet are to your pelvis, the deeper the stretch in your hips and inner thighs.

4. Allow your entire body to relax, releasing any tension in your muscles.

5. Take slow and deep breaths, allowing your breath to guide you deeper into the pose and further relax your body.

6. Remain in Reclining Bound Angle Pose for 1 to 5 minutes, or as long as feels comfortable and beneficial to you.

7. To release the pose, gently bring your knees back together and extend your legs straight out.

8. Hug your knees into your chest and gently rock from side to side to release any tension in your lower back.

9. Finally, extend your legs out straight on the mat and relax in Savasana or Corpse Pose for a few moments, allowing your body and mind to integrate the effects of the pose.

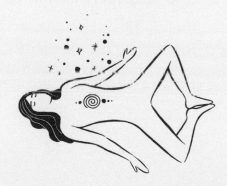

SAVASANA OR CORPSE POSE

1 Lying down on your yoga mat or a comfortable surface with your legs extended straight out in front of you, allow your feet to relax and fall open naturally.

2 Let your arms rest alongside your body, palms facing up. Keep your arms relaxed and slightly away from your torso.

3 Gently tuck your chin slightly toward your chest, lengthening the back of your neck. Ensure your head is in a comfortable and neutral position.

4 Take a moment to scan your body and release any tension. Soften your facial muscles, relax your shoulders, and let go of any tightness in your hands and feet.

5 Close your eyes to turn your focus inward and create a sense of relaxation and stillness.

6 Allow your breath to flow naturally without any effort or control. Notice the gentle rise and fall of your abdomen as you breathe.

7 Remain in this pose for 5 to 10 minutes, or longer if you have the time and desire to do so. Use this time to relax deeply and let go of any physical or mental tension.

8 When you are ready to end the pose, gently bring awareness back to your breath and your body. Begin to wiggle your fingers and toes, slowly awakening your body.

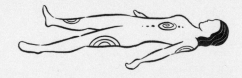

9   Bend your knees and gently roll to your right side, using your right arm as a pillow. Take a few breaths here to ease back into wakefulness.

10 When you feel ready, press your left hand into the floor and use your right hand to help you slowly sit up into a comfortable seated position.

Note Savasana or Corpse Pose is a time for deep relaxation and integration, allowing your body and mind to absorb the benefits of your yoga practice. It is an essential part of any yoga routine and is a wonderful way to end your practice on a peaceful and centred note. As with any yoga pose, listen to your body, and make any adjustments needed to ensure your comfort during Savasana.

Ground yourself with the Spinal Reset series when you are feeling tired, overworked or stressed. This practice helps you connect with your energy levels and gives you the space to explore tensions and stresses in your body, hopefully letting them go as you work through the series. Working systematically and somatically with the movement will centre you in the present with the gentle movements of the body and breath, ultimately bringing a sense of calm and presence.

Take the Plunge

So far, we've explored how to find our joy in movement and some of the science behind why different forms of movement can be so effective for us. We've delved into a few different practices, spent time reflecting, and built-up a blueprint to help us solidify our habits.

I will make a quick note here on deepening your practice, whatever your movement choice may be.

First, though, what is your response to the following statement:

Deepening your practice is not about running harder or faster, it's not about being able to do a handstand or swim for miles. It's about challenging yourself to move beyond your thinking, to explore and connect with your practice in a way that brings you new possibilities.

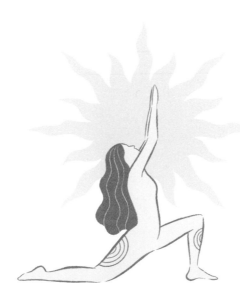

When I first arrived in India to train to teach yoga, I had a preconception that the goal was to be as thin and flexible as possible. Much of the advertising world would also have you believe this ideal. What I found, however, was my teacher Jaggi, who insisted that the goal was to be able to sit comfortably for meditation, to be healthy of mind and soul. It completely changed my thinking.

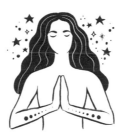

At its core, yoga is about union – aligning the mind, body and breath to achieve a harmonious state of balance and vitality. However, this union doesn't occur overnight. Rather, it unfolds gradually, requiring patience, dedication, and a willingness to explore both the physical and spiritual dimensions of the practice.

Beyond the physical poses, a deeper yoga practice often involves delving into meditation and mindfulness. This heightened self-awareness can lead to transformative shifts in one's perspective and behaviour.

Progressively deepening your yoga practice is a transformative journey that extends beyond the physical poses. It encompasses a commitment to self-awareness, mental clarity, and spiritual growth. This journey is not about reaching a destination; rather, it's about embracing the lessons learned along the way.

This view is not just limited to yoga, though; we can see the pattern here for any practice. There is an element of refining the physical, but as discussed previously, there is room in any practice for the mental and spiritual growth we so often associate with yoga.

Running for instance is more than just a physical activity – it's a way to challenge yourself, push your limits, and connect with your body and mind on a deeper level. Whether you're a casual jogger or an aspiring marathoner, there are numerous ways to progressively deepen your ability to run and unlock new levels of performance, endurance, and personal growth.

One of the fundamental principles in deepening your running ability is consistency. Regular practice builds not only physical strength and endurance but also mental resilience. Starting with a manageable routine and gradually increasing your mileage and intensity allows your body to adapt and become more efficient at running. Consistency helps solidify the habit of running, making it a part of your lifestyle rather than just a sporadic activity.

To go further in your running journey, mental fortitude is just as important as physical strength. Long runs and challenging workouts can test your mental resilience, pushing you to confront discomfort and self-doubt. Developing strategies such as positive self-talk, visualization, and mindfulness can help you stay focused and motivated, even when the going gets tough.

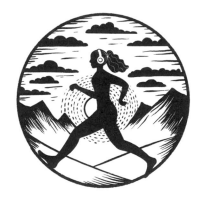

Setting goals is a powerful way to deepen your running ability. Goals provide direction and purpose to your training, giving you a tangible target to work towards. Whether it's completing a specific distance, achieving a personal best time, or conquering a challenging race, setting both short-term and long-term goals keeps you motivated and committed to your running journey. You can check out the Beginning to Run: a Guide that follows to help you get started.

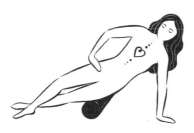

Listening to your body and prioritizing recovery is a vital aspect of deepening your running ability. Overtraining can lead to burnout and injuries. Incorporating rest days, foam rolling, stretching, and adequate sleep into your routine promotes physical and mental rejuvenation, allowing your body to adapt and grow stronger.

Ultimately, deepening your ability to run is an ongoing process that encompasses physical, mental and emotional growth. It's a journey that requires dedication, patience, and a willingness to step out of your comfort zone. With consistent practice, proper training, mental resilience, goal setting, and a focus on recovery, you can unlock new levels of performance, personal achievement, and a deeper connection with yourself through the art of running.

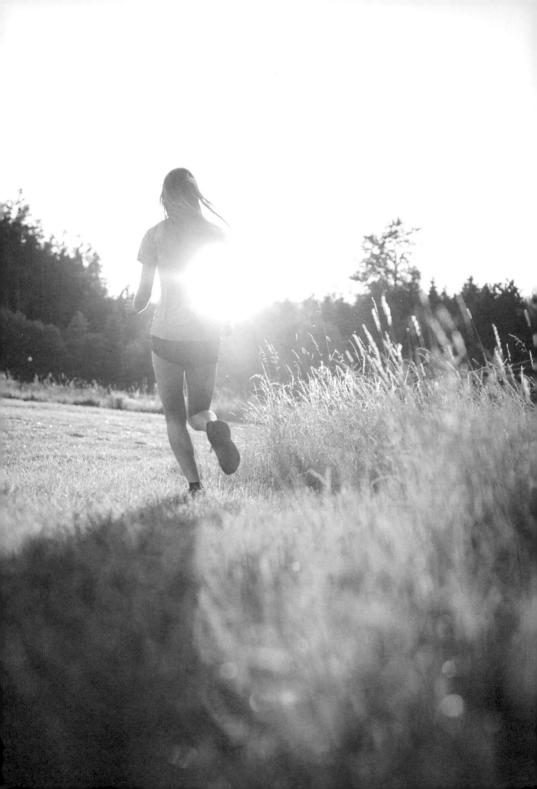

Beginning To Run: a Guide

Whether you are a complete beginner or have dabbled somewhat in running, this guide is to help you begin your running journey, find consistency and teach you how to mix up your training to avoid plateaus and prevent overuse injuries. Incorporating different types of runs, such as long runs, tempo runs, intervals and hill training, challenges your body in various ways. The following guide will help you over the course of 12 weeks to train to easily manage a 10k run or race.

REMEMBER:

Deepening your running ability also involves paying attention to proper form and technique. Running with proper posture, efficient arm movement and a balanced stride can significantly improve your performance and reduce the risk of injury.

Similarly, nutrition and hydration play a crucial role in enhancing your running performance. Fuelling your body with the right nutrients before, during, and after your runs can improve your energy levels, endurance and recovery. Staying hydrated ensures that your body functions optimally and helps prevent the onset of fatigue during your runs.

For more information on supporting your body for running, whether that's improving your technique or nutrition and hydration, please see the sources I recommend in the Further Reading section at the end of this book.

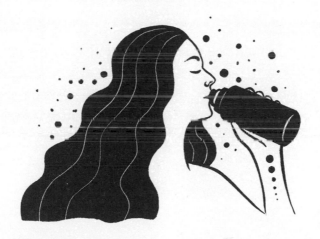

ACTIVITY: 12 WEEKS TO 10K

Use the following plan as starting point, scheduling your runs for alternate days with a rest day between, and adding in an extra day of cross-training such as swimming or cycling or yoga in each week. Don't forget to stretch before and after your runs, and monitor your breathing.

A NOTE ABOUT PACE

› Easy pace – This should feel like a comfortable, slightly out of breath pace. You could hold light conversation if needed.

› Long pace – Slightly slower than easy pace, this is a pace you could maintain for a long period of time and hold conversation easily while running.

› Tempo runs – These are faster runs at 'short race' pace (perhaps 5k race pace), and should feel breathy! Aim to run at the speed required to complete your 'race' (or the chosen distance you are ultimately aiming for) in your target finish time.

› Interval runs – Quick stop/start sprints mixed with walking/slower running.

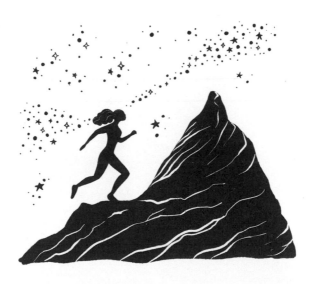

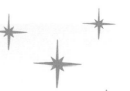

WEEK 1–4: BUILDING BASE ENDURANCE

Day 1: Easy pace, 15–20 minute run, out and back
Day 2: Long pace, 30 minutes (in the first week or two try to run
as much as possible in this half hour but take walking rests if
necessary, aim to build up to running the whole 30 minutes)
Day 3: Tempo run, 1 mile (1.6k) at the speed required for your target time
(see A Note About Pace). Use this run as a measure of progress.

WEEK 5–8: INCREASING ENDURANCE

Day 1: Intervals, 30–40 minutes walk/run or run/sprint
Day 2: Easy pace, 5k (3 mile) run
Day 3: Tempo run, 1 mile, as weeks 1–4 (use as a measure of progress).

WEEK 9-12: ADDING LONGER RUNS

Day 1: Long pace, 40–50 minutes, and try to include a hill or other terrain.
Day 2: Tempo run, 5k at the speed required for your
target time (use as a measure of progress).
Day 3: Easy pace, 50–60 minutes

10K TEST WEEK

Day 1: Easy pace, 30 minutes
Day 2: Intervals, 20 minutes
Day 3: Very light cross-training

TEST DAY: CONGRATULATIONS!

Run your 10k route and enjoy the experience.

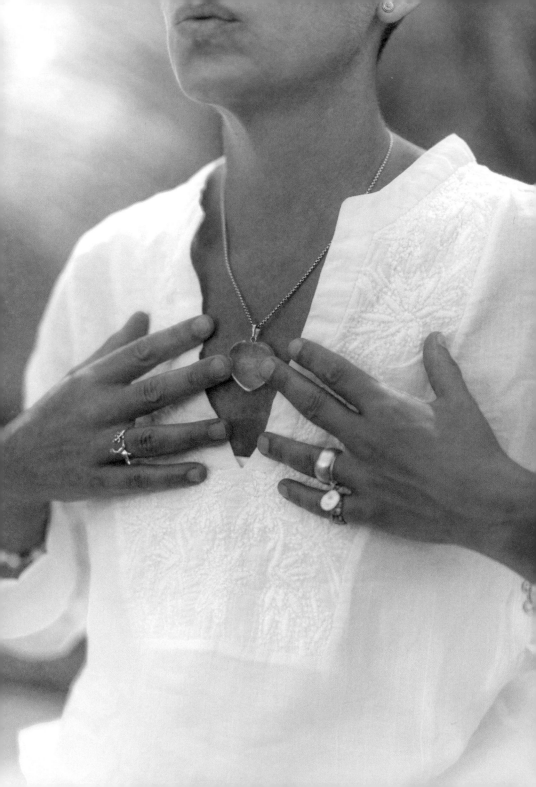

CHAPTER 2
Move with Your Breath

"Feelings come and go like clouds in a windy sky. Conscious breathing is my anchor."

Thich Nhat Hanh, Bhuddist monk, peace activist, teacher and author

Stop for a moment and consider, how do you breathe? Through your nose, mouth? What are you doing right now? Are your breaths deep, short, longer on the exhale?

Breathwork and the idea of regulating and expanding breathing and discovering techniques to do this is something that is becoming more mainstream. When I first started teaching yoga, nearly ten years ago, it was very much the strange five minutes or so added on at the end in a typically western yoga class. Yet it is one of the fundamental processes for enhancing any movement or meditation practice. In this section we are going to explore some of the science behind breathing and some of the foundational practices you can do to improve your lung capacity, calm your nervous system and increase that connection between mind, body and breath.

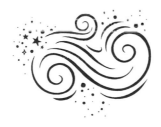

Breathing Fundamentals

Breathing is an involuntary action that sustains our lives from the moment we are born. Beyond its essential role in supplying oxygen to our cells and expelling carbon dioxide, the science of breathing, known as respiratory physiology, reveals a complex interplay of physiological processes that influence our overall health, mental wellbeing, and even athletic performance.

THE SCIENCE OF BREATHING: UNVEILING THE POWER OF RESPIRATION

At the core of breathing lies the respiratory system, a network of organs including the lungs, diaphragm, and various muscles that work in harmony to facilitate the exchange of gases. Inhalation brings oxygen-rich air into the lungs, where oxygen diffuses into the bloodstream and is carried to cells for energy production. Simultaneously, carbon dioxide, a waste product, is transported from the cells back to the lungs and expelled during exhalation.

However, the science of breathing goes beyond basic gas exchange. Research has unveiled the profound impact of breathing patterns on our physiological and psychological states. The autonomic nervous system, which controls involuntary bodily functions, is divided into two branches: the sympathetic nervous system (SNS) and the parasympathetic nervous system (PNS). Deep, slow breathing activates the PNS, promoting relaxation, lowered heart rate, and reduced stress levels. On the other hand, rapid, shallow breathing triggers the SNS, leading to heightened alertness and the 'fight or flight' response.

Conscious control of breathing, often associated with practices like meditation and yoga, allows individuals to regulate their physiological responses. Techniques such as diaphragmatic breathing, where the breath originates from the belly rather than shallow chest breathing, can induce a calming effect, lower blood pressure, and improve overall emotional wellbeing. In yoga this is often known as 'deep yogic breathing'. Using the guide in the following activity take a moment to have a go and practice breathing this way. What do you notice? Do you naturally breathe this way or is this something new?

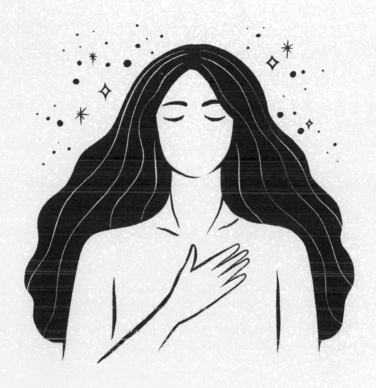

ACTIVITY: DEEP YOGIC BREATHING

1. Find a comfortable position.
Sit or lie down in a comfortable position. You can sit with your legs crossed or lie on your back with knees bent and feet flat on the floor. Place your hands on your abdomen to feel the movement.

2. Relax your body.
Close your eyes or gaze at a fixed point and take a moment to relax your body. Soften your facial muscles, release tension in your shoulders, and let go of any tightness in your jaw or neck.

3. Inhale through the nose.
Take a slow and deep breath in through your nose. Feel the air moving through your nostrils and into your lungs.

4. Expand your belly.
As you inhale, focus on expanding your belly outward. Allow your diaphragm to descend, which creates space for your lungs to fill with air. Feel your abdomen rise as you inhale.

5. Feel the fullness.
Continue to inhale deeply until you feel your lungs and lower ribcage expanding fully. Keep your chest relatively still, allowing the breath to fill the lower part of your lungs.

6. Exhale through the nose.
Exhale slowly and completely through your nose. Feel your belly gently contract as you expel the air.

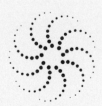

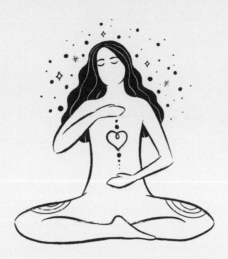

7. Empty your lungs.
Empty your lungs completely by contracting your abdominal muscles slightly at the end of the exhale.

8. Maintain a smooth rhythm.
Begin to establish a smooth and rhythmic pattern of breathing. Inhale deeply and slowly, filling your belly and lower lungs, and then exhale slowly and completely.

9. Stay present.
Focus your attention on the breath throughout the practice. If your mind wanders, gently bring your focus back to the sensation of the breath in your abdomen.

10. Practice mindful breathing.
As you continue the Deep Yogic Breathing, use it as a tool for mindfulness and relaxation. Observe how your body responds to the breath and let go of any tension or stress with each exhale.

Hopefully, you noticed a sense of quiet and calm descending upon you. Deep Yogic Breathing is a simple yet powerful technique that can be practiced anywhere, at any time, to promote a sense of calm and relaxation. Regular practice of this breathing technique can help reduce stress, lower blood pressure, and improve overall wellbeing. It's a foundational aspect of many yoga and meditation practices, and it serves as a gateway to deeper states of awareness and inner peace.

BREATHING FOR MOVEMENT

In recent years, the science of breathing has extended its reach into the world of sports and fitness. Athletes and trainers recognise the potential of optimised breathing techniques to enhance performance. Breath control during exercise can improve oxygen delivery to muscles, delay fatigue and regulate heart rate. Techniques like 'paced breathing', where the rhythm of inhalation and exhalation is synchronised with movement, have enhanced endurance and overall athletic output. This naturally happens in yoga, but it can also be applied to any physical movement, such as running, swimming, climbing or hiking.

BREATHING FOR WELLBEING

The connection between breathing and various health conditions is another avenue of scientific exploration. Conditions such as asthma, sleep apnoea, and chronic obstructive pulmonary disease (COPD) are directly related to respiratory function. Understanding breathing mechanics could lead to improved treatments and therapies for these ailments.

Furthermore, the connection between breathing and mental health is garnering increased attention. Research suggests that specific breathing patterns can influence mood, anxiety and cognitive function. For instance, deep and rhythmic breathing can alleviate symptoms of anxiety and depression by modulating neurotransmitter release and promoting a sense of calm.

Yoga has recognised the value of conscious breathing practices for centuries; in the next section, we will take a deeper look at some of these ancient traditions and consider how we can incorporate them into our everyday.

Deepening Your Practice

Throughout history, the practice of pranayama has been guided by the principle that the breath serves as a bridge between the physical body and the subtle energies of the mind and spirit. Different yogic lineages have developed various pranayama techniques (*prana* roughly meaning life force and *yama* meaning knowledge of), each with its own approach and emphasis. These techniques focus on controlling and harnessing the breath to achieve various physical, mental and spiritual benefits. The history of pranayama and its evolution within the broader context of yoga can be traced through different periods.

VEDIC PERIOD (1500–500BCE)

The earliest mentions of breath control practices can be found in the Vedas, the ancient sacred texts of India. Pranayama was introduced as a way to control the life force, prana, and was associated with the regulation of vital energies.

UPANISHAD PERIOD (800–400BCE)

The Upanishads elaborated on the concept of prana and introduced the idea of prana as the universal energy that permeates all living beings. Breathing practices were considered a means to control the mind and attain higher states of consciousness.

CLASSICAL YOGA PERIOD (200BCE–500CE)

The *Yoga Sutras of Patanjali*, a foundational text of classical yoga, mentions pranayama as a vital practice to control the fluctuations of the mind (*chitta vrittis*). Patanjali's approach emphasised the integration of pranayama within the eightfold path of yoga, including ethical guidelines, physical postures and meditation.

HATHA YOGA PERIOD (9TH–15TH CENTURY)

The Hatha yoga tradition gave rise to a more systematic exploration of pranayama techniques. Texts like the *Hatha Yoga Pradipika* and the *Gheranda Samhita* introduced detailed instructions on various pranayama practices, emphasizing purification of the energy channels (*nadis*) and awakening of spiritual energies (*kundalini*).

MODERN PERIOD (19TH CENTURY–PRESENT)

In the late 19th and early 20th centuries, yoga experienced a revival and began to gain popularity in the West. Influential figures like Swami Vivekananda and Paramahamsa Yogananda introduced pranayama practices to western audiences, contributing to the integration of breath control techniques into yoga teachings outside of India.

Pranayama breathing techniques

Some well-known pranayama techniques include:

ANULOMA VILLOMA (Alternate Nostril Breathing)

Involves alternating breath between the nostrils to balance the energy flow and harmonise the body and mind.

UJJAYI PRANAYAMA (Ocean Breath)

Characterised by a soft hissing sound produced by slight throat constriction during inhalation and exhalation. It promotes relaxation and concentration during asana yoga practice.

BHASTRIKA PRANAYAMA (Bellows Breath)

A vigorous breathing technique involving rapid and forceful inhalations and exhalations. It energises the body and clears the mind.

Another more recent technique you may see in yoga classes is 'four-part' or 'square breath' which promotes relaxation and concentrated awareness. Tips on how to practice both alternate nostril breathing and four-part breath are included here for you to practice at your own leisure, I recommend journalling and reflecting on the practices to help you increase your awareness.

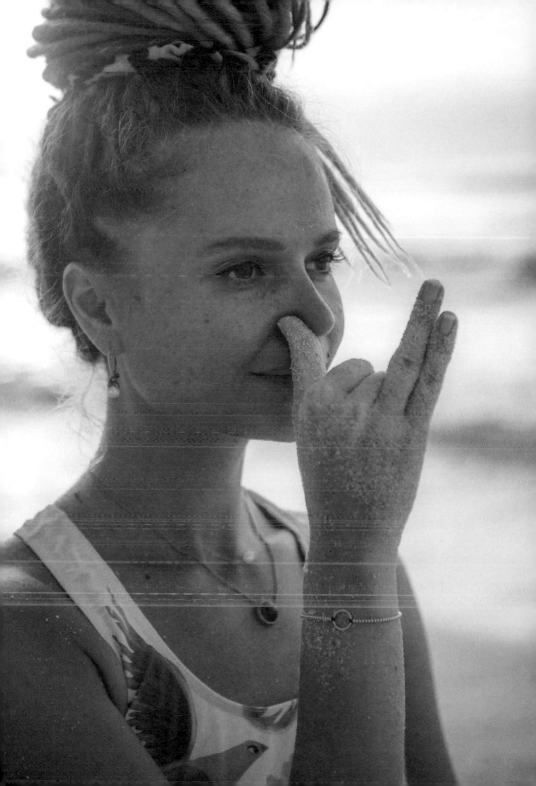

ACTIVITY: ALTERNATE NOSTRIL BREATHING

Alternate Nostril Breathing, also known as Nadi Shodhana or Anuloma Villoma pranayama in yoga, is a powerful breathing technique that helps balance the flow of energy in the body and calm the mind. It involves using the thumb and fingers to close and open the nostrils alternately while breathing. Here's how to practice Alternate Nostril Breathing:

1. Find a comfortable seated position.
Sit in a comfortable cross-legged position on the floor or on a chair with your spine straight and shoulders relaxed. You can also practice this technique lying down if sitting is uncomfortable.

2. Rest your left hand.
Place your left hand on your left knee, palm facing up, in the Chin Mudra (index finger and thumb touching). This mudra symbolises unity and consciousness.

3. Nasagra Mudra with your right hand.
Use your right hand to perform the Nasagra Mudra. To do this softly press your index and middle fingers to your palm, leaving your thumb, ring finger, and little finger extended.

4. Begin with an exhale.
Close your right nostril with your right thumb, and exhale completely through your left nostril. Gently contract your abdominal muscles to expel the breath fully.

5. Inhale through your left nostril.
Keeping the right nostril closed, inhale slowly and deeply through your left nostril. Feel the breath filling your lungs and expanding your abdomen.

6. Close your left nostril.
Close your left nostril with your right ring finger and little finger, and simultaneously release the right nostril.

7. Exhale through your right nostril.
Exhale completely through your right nostril. Feel the breath leaving your body and the abdomen contracting.

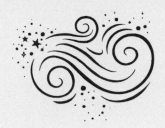

8. Inhale through your right nostril.
Inhale deeply and slowly through your right nostril while keeping the left nostril closed.

9. Close your right nostril.
Close your right nostril with your right thumb and release the left nostril.

10. Exhale through your left nostril.
Exhale completely through your left nostril.

11. Continue the pattern.
This completes one round of Alternate Nostril Breathing. Continue this pattern of inhaling through one nostril, switching, and exhaling through the other nostril for several rounds. You can start with 5 to 10 rounds and gradually increase the number as you feel comfortable.

12. Finish with your left nostril.
To end the practice, complete the final exhale through your left nostril and release your right hand back to rest on your left knee. Take a few normal breaths, observing the sensations in your body and mind.

Alternate Nostril Breathing is a balancing and calming pranayama technique that harmonises the flow of energy (*prana*) in the body and helps clear the energy channels (*nadis*). It is an excellent practice for reducing stress, promoting mental clarity and preparing the mind for meditation. As with all pranayama practices, practice with mindfulness and ease, avoiding any strain or forceful breathing.

ACTIVITY: FOUR-PART BREATH

The Four-part Breath, also known as square breathing or box breathing, is a simple and effective breathing technique used to promote relaxation, reduce stress, and increase focus and concentration. It involves equalizing the duration of the inhalation, holding the breath, exhalation, and holding the breath again, creating a square-like pattern. Here's how to practice the Four-part Breath:

1. Find a comfortable position.
Sit in a comfortable position with your spine straight and shoulders relaxed. You can sit cross-legged on the floor or on a chair, or you can practice this technique lying down.

2. Nasagra Mudra with your right hand.
Use your right hand to perform the Nasagra Mudra, just like in the Alternate Nostril Breathing activity. Softly press your index and middle fingers to your palm, leaving your thumb, ring finger and little finger extended.

3. Inhale to the count of four.
Begin by inhaling slowly and deeply through your nose to the count of four. Feel the breath filling your lungs and expanding your abdomen.

4. Hold your breath to the count of four.
Once you've completed the inhalation, hold your breath for the same count of four. Keep your lungs and abdomen comfortably filled with air during this breath-holding phase.

5. Exhale to the count of four.
Begin exhaling slowly and completely through your nose to the count of four. Empty your lungs and feel your abdomen contract.

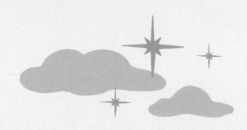

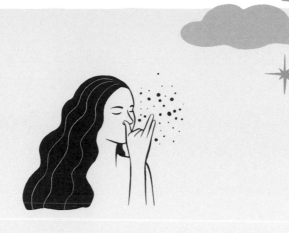

6. Hold your breath (with empty lungs) to the count of four.

After completing the exhale, hold your breath again for the same count of four before starting the next inhalation.

7. Repeat the pattern.

This completes one round of the Four-part Breath. Continue this pattern of inhaling, holding, exhaling and holding again for several rounds. Start with 5 to 10 rounds and gradually increase the number as you feel comfortable.

8. Maintain a smooth rhythm.

Focus on maintaining a smooth and steady rhythm throughout the practice. The duration of each phase (inhale, hold, exhale, hold) should be the same, creating the square-like pattern

9. Relax and observe.

After completing the rounds, release the breath control and breathe naturally. Take a moment to observe the effects of the Four-part Breath on your body and mind. Notice any sensations of relaxation or increased mental clarity.

The Four-part Breath is a powerful technique to help regulate the autonomic nervous system, promoting a sense of calm and balance. It can be used as a standalone practice for relaxation or as a preparation for meditation and mindfulness exercises. As with any breathwork, if you feel any discomfort or dizziness, return to normal breathing and try again later with shorter counts or fewer rounds. The Four-part Breath can be done anywhere and at any time to bring about a sense of peace and centredness.

Applying Breathwork to Movement

As mentioned before, there are many advantages to applying conscious breathwork to your movement. Some of the benefits include:

> Increased oxygenation and energy

> Efficient waste removal of carbon dioxide

> Stress reduction, particularly in hormone responses

> Increased focus and concentration

> Optimised performance due to consistent rhythm and effective pacing

> Reduced muscle tension

> Increased body awareness and mind-body connection

> Effective recovery and cool down

> Enhanced mental state

So how can we apply these breathing practices to our movement patterns? The following are a few quick examples of how to use breath effectively in yoga, running and cold-water swimming.

YOGA

Using your breath to regulate holds in yoga is a fundamental aspect of maintaining a balanced and effective practice. The breath serves as a guiding force that helps you stay present, manage discomfort, and promote relaxation during static yoga poses. You can use your breath to regulate holds in different yoga postures by focusing on even breathing, lengthening your exhalations, breath counting and synchronising breath to flow of movement. Finally, by using diaphragmatic breathing you can increase recovery in Savasana or the rest at the end of physical practice.

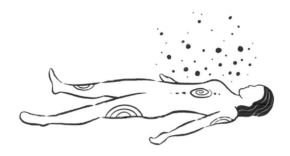

RUNNING

Breathing is not only essential for providing oxygen to your muscles but also plays a role in maintaining a steady rhythm and managing your energy levels, both of which will improve your running performance. A few ideas you could try while running are practicing nasal breathing, matching breath to stride, focusing on deep breathing or rhythmic breathing and using your breath to regulate or lessen 'panting' on hills. If you find you struggle to breathe entirely nasally whilst running, focus on inhaling through your nose and out through your mouth.

Finally, pay attention to how different breathing techniques affect your running performance and comfort. The key is to find a breathing rhythm that suits your pace, terrain and individual preferences. By incorporating mindful and intentional breathing techniques, you can optimise your running experience and achieve better results.

COLD WATER IMMERSION

Did you know that for centuries yoga practitioners and Tibetan monks have been utilising the breathing techniques popularised by modern extreme athletes to perform incredible feats of cold water immersion?

Cold water immersion is something that either terrifies or excites people. It is considered a practice of mental and physical resilience and can be a challenge to master. There are incredible benefits to cold water immersion including:

> Improved circulation and blood flow

> Enhanced immune function and reduced inflammation

> Boosted metabolism and increased fat burning

> Reduced stress, anxiety and improved mental clarity

> Enhanced focus and concentration

> Faster recovery for athletes and reduced muscle soreness

Breathing effectively during cold water immersion is essential to manage the initial shock, maintain control, and support your body's response to the cold. Controlled breathing can help reduce the body's stress response, prevent hyperventilation, and improve your overall comfort in cold water. This control stems mainly from your ability to regulate your exhalation. There is more on this in the Guide to Cold Water Immersion that follows.

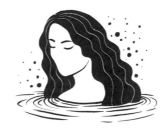

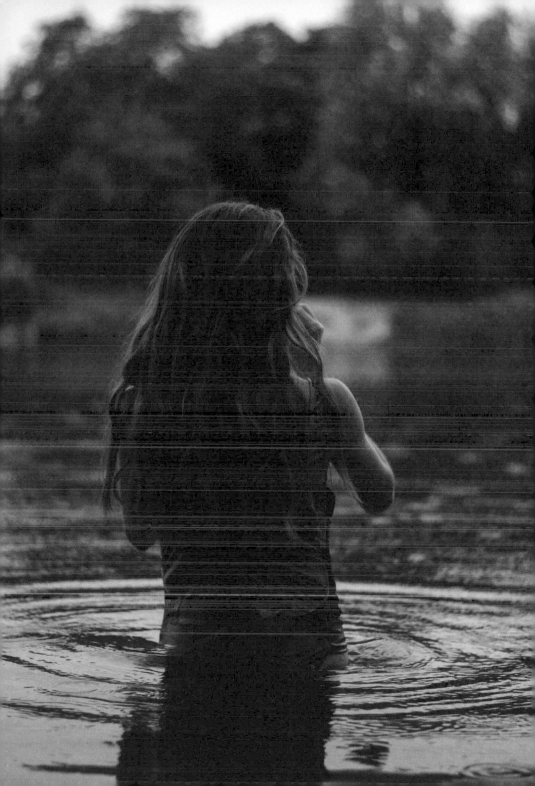

ACTIVITY: GUIDE TO COLD WATER IMMERSION

Cold water immersion, also known as cold water therapy or cold plunges, is the practice of submerging your body in cold water for therapeutic and health benefits. When combined with breathwork it can have additional physiological and psychological effects.

Here are my top tips to starting your cold water immersion journey:

BEFORE STARTING

› Consult with a healthcare professional if you are in any way unsure about your capacity to undertake the practice.

› Choose the right location: a cold plunge pool, your shower or a calm body of water such as a tarn or small lake. Take extra precautions if practising outdoors, such as going with a confident group, being able to swim and choosing somewhere close enough for access to help if needed.

› Choose appropriate gear such as neoprene gloves and boots, or even a full suit.

› Start gradually using the tips below.

COLD WATER IMMERSION

› Prepare your body with a small, dynamic warm-up.

› Regulate your breath before entering (see Deep Yogic Breathing).

› Enter the water slowly.

› Focus on slow controlled exhalations during your immersion.

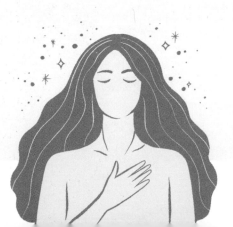

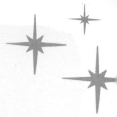

AFTER COLD WATER IMMERSION

› Exit gradually to avoid a shock response.

› Warm up immediately with towels and easy to put on layers. If outdoors I like to bring warm water bottles to place in my layers and something warm for my feet to stand on.

› Continue breathwork.

› Hydrate and nourish with a warm drink and cake (or other alternative).

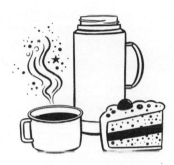

IMPORTANT CONSIDERATIONS

› Always listen to your body and avoid overexertion or prolonged cold water immersion. A few minutes gradually building up to longer periods is safest.

› Cold water immersion is not recommended for individuals with certain medical conditions, so consult your healthcare provider before starting the practice.

› If you experience any adverse reactions or discomfort during cold water immersion, stop immediately and seek medical attention if necessary.

› Gradually build up your tolerance to cold water immersion over time.

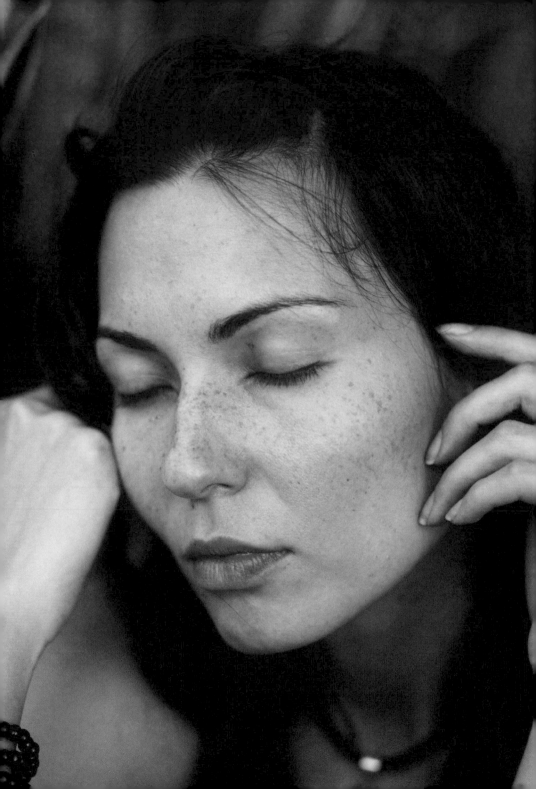

CHAPTER 3

Move with Your Mind

"Quiet the mind, and the soul will speak."

Ma Jaya Sati Bhagavati, Hindu spiritual teacher and author

So far, we've delved into how we redefine our relationship with movement, we've built up practices to incorporate our breath, and now we are going to solidify our understanding by looking at the power of our minds in relation to building new habits.

Have you ever wondered why habits can feel hard to build? Do you check your self-limiting thoughts at the door of building a new practice? Have you accumulated the tools to help protect your mind from feeling like it will fail every time you face a challenge in your practice? This final section of the book is designed to increase your understanding about how our minds work and the practices that can help bolster your resilience, mindfulness and compassion for yourself. As you read each section, keeping a diary and trying to reflect on key questions that arise might be helpful to your ongoing journey to a more holistic and healing movement practice.

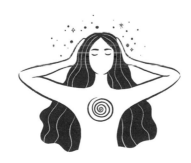

Mind-science

As with the body, it is helpful to understand how reflective, flexible and resilient our minds can be. Biological, psychological, environmental and social factors affect our mental development, and here we'll delve into the science behind it all. As you read each section, try to reflect on the key question and use it to help you build an overall picture of your mental resilience.

BUILDING RESILIENCE

Resilience is the ability of individuals, communities, or systems to adapt, recover and thrive in the face of significant challenges. It is rooted in various scientific factors, such as psychology, biology and social sciences.

Resilience can be influenced by numerous natural biological factors, including genetics, brain structure and function, and the body's stress response system. For example, certain genetic variations can affect an individual's sensitivity to stress-related disorders, while a well-regulated stress response system can help individuals bounce back from difficult situations.

How do you normally respond to stressful situations? Fight, flight, freeze or fawn?
Fight normally presents as facing a perceived threat with aggression, flight inherently implies running away, freeze is becoming inert in the face of danger, and fawn often results in attempting to please to avoid conflict. You may be a mix of all or some of these.

Similarly, psychological factors play a crucial role in resilience. Cognitive processes such as positive thinking, problem-solving skills, self-efficacy (belief in one's ability to overcome challenges), and emotional regulation contribute to an individual's ability to cope with adversity. Having a sense of purpose, setting achievable goals, and cultivating optimism can also enhance resilience.

What goals have you set recently that were successful, and why do you think you achieved them?
Goals may be small achievable tasks, deadlines at work, building a new routine or habit or simply getting on with a long-awaited job. They can be whatever you feel a sense of achievement from.

Social connections and support networks are also essential for resilience. Strong social bonds like family, friends and communities provide emotional support, practical assistance and a sense of belonging. The presence of supportive relationships can buffer the impact of stressors and provide resources for individuals to navigate challenging situations.

Who are the people in your key, supportive relationships, and how do they buffer the impact of stressors? List them.
Consider family members, close friends and supportive colleagues. Do they offer an ear, help problem-solve, or give sage advice? In what ways do you feel they support you the most?

Resilience involves adaptability and flexibility in change. This includes being open to new ideas, adjusting goals or strategies when needed, and embracing uncertainty. Flexibility allows individuals to respond creatively and effectively to challenges, promoting resilience.

What three new ideas have you discovered in the last month, and how did they change your perception?
Maybe these are new ways of doing a routine you've always done, or a new piece of information or perspective you've never considered.

Learning and growth are often a part of becoming more resilient. Through experiences of adversity, individuals can develop new skills, gain insights, and develop a deeper understanding of themselves and the world around them. This growth mindset enables individuals to approach future challenges with increased confidence and adaptability.

What experience do you feel has made you the most resilient? Describe a key moment or challenge that changed you.
This can be from any period in your life – something positive or negative – where you feel there was a key moment of learning that increased your capacity to grow mentally.

Lastly, individuals' physical and social environments can influence their resilience. Factors such as access to resources, socioeconomic status, community support, and exposure to violence or trauma can impact an individual's ability to cope with, and recover from, adversity. Creating supportive and nurturing environments can foster resilience in individuals and communities.

Where do you feel a sense of community most?
Are you part of any groups or bands, or community activities? Maybe you help at a charity or are involved in a religious organisation?

It's important to note that resilience is not a fixed trait but a dynamic process that can be cultivated and strengthened. By understanding the underlying scientific principles, we can develop strategies and systems that promote resilience in ourselves.

NEUROPLASTICITY IN A NUTSHELL

A barrier to our growth is the idea that, as adults, we have no time to pick up something new. Doubts fill our minds with negative, self-deprecating voices that tell us we can't join a drumming band or develop the ability to play a sport we may have failed at school. There is a myth that once we pass a certain age, our learning is 'done'; however, that is not the case.

Neuroplasticity refers to the brain's ability to change and reorganise its structure, function and connections in response to experiences, learning and environmental influences. In itself, 'plasticity' refers to the brain's malleability and capacity to adapt and reshape itself throughout a person's life. Research into this pliability suggests that although there are 'critical' periods of development in which the brain is at its most malleable, there is no real limit to learning; lifelong learning can keep us more mentally and physically flexible for longer!

We tend to think about changes in the brain happening during those critical periods of development, which are characterised by heightened neuroplasticity. The brain is susceptible to specific environmental inputs and experiences during these periods. For instance, early childhood is a critical period for language acquisition, and the brain exhibits heightened plasticity during this time, allowing children to learn language more effortlessly.

However, there are other key ways in which the brain changes over time:

Firstly, structural plasticity involves changes in the brain's physical structure, such as the growth of new neurons (neurogenesis), and the remodelling of existing connections. Structural changes can occur in response to learning, environmental enrichment and experiences.

Functional plasticity refers to the brain's ability to redistribute and reorganise functions in response to input, damage or learning changes. For example, if a particular brain area becomes damaged, other regions may assume its operations, leading to functional reorganisation.

Similarly, synaptic plasticity involves changes in the strength and efficacy of synaptic connections between neurons. It is a fundamental mechanism underlying learning, memory formation and adaptive responses. Synaptic plasticity allows synapses to strengthen or weaken based on patterns of neural activity.

Another factor by which neuroplasticity is heavily influenced is experience and environmental factors. The brain constantly adapts and remodels itself based on the sensory input, learning and experiences an individual encounters. For example, learning a new skill, playing a musical instrument, or acquiring new knowledge can lead to structural and functional changes in the brain that support acquiring and retaining that skill or expertise.

By understanding these different factors, we can begin unpicking how to promote and strengthen neuroplasticity. Engaging in activities that challenge the brain and provide new learning experiences can enhance the brain's ability to adapt and rewire itself.

Ways to Strengthen Neuroplasticity

› In order to strengthen these developments in the brain we can look at several different ways to engage our brains and ensure continual growth.

› For instance, engaging in lifelong learning and academic activities can promote neuroplasticity. This can include reading, solving puzzles, learning a new language, playing musical instruments, or participating in mentally stimulating hobbies. These activities keep the brain active, challenge cognitive abilities, and encourage the formation of new neural connections.

› Another way to enhance neuroplasticity is regular physical activity. Aerobic exercises like running, swimming or cycling positively affect brain health and plasticity. Exercise increases blood flow to the brain, promotes the release of growth factors, and stimulates the production of new neurons and synaptic connections.

› Similarly, mindfulness practices and meditation have been found to promote neuroplasticity. These techniques involve focused attention, awareness of the present moment, and non-judgmental acceptance. Regular mindfulness and meditation can strengthen neural connections, improve emotional regulation, and enhance cognitive functions.

> Likewise, meaningful social interactions can also positively impact brain plasticity. Engaging in conversations, building relationships, and participating in group activities stimulate cognitive processes and emotional wellbeing. Social support and connection also contribute to resilience and can help buffer against the negative effects of stress on the brain.

> Something less thought about in terms of developing neuroplasticity is exposure to new and stimulating environments. Novelty activates the brain's reward system, releases neurotransmitters like dopamine, and encourages the formation of new connections. Exploring new places, engaging in new activities, and seeking diverse experiences can all contribute to neuroplasticity.

> Taking care of your overall health promotes neuroplasticity. This includes maintaining a balanced diet rich in nutrients, staying adequately hydrated, managing stress levels, and avoiding harmful substances such as excessive alcohol or drug use. Sufficient sleep and rest are also essential for optimal brain function and neuroplasticity. During sleep, the brain consolidates memories, clears out waste products, and allows synaptic pruning and reorganisation. Getting quality sleep regularly supports neuroplasticity and cognitive performance.

> It's worth noting that individual differences in neuroplasticity exist, and the extent to which neuroplastic changes occur varies among individuals. However, incorporating these strategies into your lifestyle can create an environment that fosters neuroplasticity, supports brain health and leads to a growth mindset.

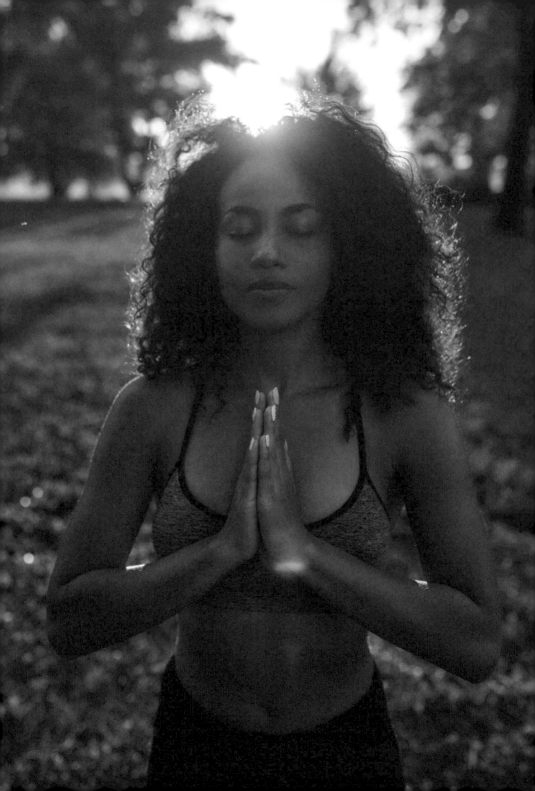

Growth Mindset

Now that we've explored the brain and the incredible ways neuroplasticity can be developed within, it is worth looking at the key scientific theorist and renowned psychologist Carol Dweck. She is best known for her groundbreaking work on growth mindset. Through extensive research, Dweck has demonstrated how individuals' beliefs about their abilities can shape their motivation, resilience and achievement.

Dweck's work on growth mindset revolves around the belief that individuals can develop their abilities and intelligence through effort, learning and perseverance. She distinguishes between a fixed mindset, where individuals believe their talents and skills are innate and unchangeable, and a growth mindset, where individuals accept that their abilities can be developed through dedication and hard work. Dweck's research shows that those with a growth mindset tend to embrace challenges, persist in the face of obstacles, and see failures as opportunities for growth. They have a more positive attitude toward learning and are likelier to achieve their full potential. Ultimately, by understanding and adopting a growth mindset, individuals can cultivate resilience, motivation, and a lifelong love for learning. Take the following Growth Mindset Quiz to see how flexible your brain is!

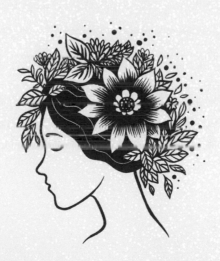

ACTIVITY: GROWTH MINDSET QUIZ

When faced with a difficult task, I believe that:

a) My abilities determine my performance.

b) My effort and perseverance can improve my performance.

Failure is:

a) A sign that I lack the necessary skills or talents.

b) An opportunity to learn and grow.

Challenges are:

a) Something to avoid or fear because they might expose my weaknesses.

b) Opportunities to stretch my abilities and develop new skills.

Feedback and criticism:

a) Threaten my self-esteem because they imply that I'm not good enough.

b) Help me identify areas for improvement and motivate me to grow.

When I encounter setbacks or obstacles, I tend to:

a) Give up easily or feel discouraged.

b) Persist and find alternative strategies to overcome them.

When others succeed, I:

a) Feel jealous or threatened because it highlights my own shortcomings.

b) Feel inspired and motivated to learn from their achievements.

I believe intelligence and talent are:

a) Fixed traits that cannot be significantly changed.

b) Capable of being developed and expanded with effort and practice.

When it comes to learning and personal growth, I:

a) Prefer to stick to what I'm already good at.

b) Embrace new challenges and continuously seek opportunities to learn and improve.

Scoring:

Count the number of 'a' and 'b' responses.

If you have more 'a' responses, it suggests a tendency towards a fixed mindset.

If you have more 'b' responses, it indicates a leaning towards a growth mindset.

Remember, this quiz provides a general indication and is not a definitive measure of your mindset. Reflecting on your beliefs and attitudes towards challenges, effort and learning is important to understand your mindset better.

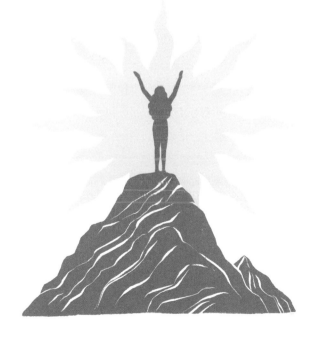

Practising Resilience

Practicing resilience involves developing the capacity to adapt, bounce back from challenges, and maintain a positive outlook in the face of adversity. Resilience is a valuable skill that can be cultivated over time through various strategies and mindset shifts. There are many ways in which to strengthen resilience in both your mindset and body. A few suggestions are:

DEVELOP A GROWTH MINDSET
› Embrace challenges as opportunities for growth and learning.
› View setbacks as temporary and believe in your ability to improve and overcome.

BUILD STRONG SOCIAL SUPPORT
› Cultivate relationships with friends, family and a support network.
› Reach out to others for help, guidance and emotional support during tough times.

PRACTICE SELF-CARE
› Prioritise your physical, mental and emotional wellbeing.
› Engage in activities that recharge and nourish you, such as exercise, hobbies and relaxation techniques.

CULTIVATE OPTIMISM
› Focus on the positive aspects of situations.
› Train your mind to find silver linings and opportunities even in difficult circumstances.

DEVELOP PROBLEM-SOLVING SKILLS
› Approach challenges with a solution-oriented mindset.
› Break down problems into manageable steps and explore different approaches.

PRACTICE MINDFULNESS AND ACCEPTANCE

> Practice mindfulness meditation to stay present and reduce stress.

> Accept that some challenges are beyond your control and focus on managing your response.

STAY FLEXIBLE AND ADAPTABLE

> Embrace change as a natural part of life.

> Adapt your plans and strategies when faced with unexpected obstacles.

SET REALISTIC GOALS

> Break down larger goals into smaller, achievable steps.

> Celebrate your progress along the way to build confidence.

SEEK PROFESSIONAL HELP WHEN NEEDED

> If facing significant challenges, consider seeking guidance from a therapist or counsellor.

> Mental health professionals can provide tools and strategies for building resilience.

PRACTICE GRATITUDE

> Focus on the positive aspects of your life and express gratitude for what you have.

> Gratitude can shift your perspective and improve your overall outlook.

LEARN FROM SETBACKS

> Reflect on past challenges and setbacks to identify lessons learned.

> Use these experiences as opportunities to gain wisdom and resilience.

ENGAGE IN ACTS OF KINDNESS

> Helping others and contributing to your community can provide a sense of purpose and fulfilment.

> Acts of kindness also strengthen your social connections.

Ways to Develop Resilience

› We are going to take a moment here to look at three aspects of developing resilience: self-care, mindfulness and gratitude. All three aspects are strengthened when we reflect on our habits and practices and consider the changes we can make to incorporate each daily. This book has hopefully given you a plethora of techniques to help you create a great basis for practising all three, however I'd like to introduce you to two more of my ultimate meditative practices to keep you inspired and on your journey to a more mindful, healing movement attitude.

› The first is a mindful body scan. I use this regularly in classes to help my students gain that subtle, intuitive insight into their bodies and appreciate the small fluctuations and changes life brings us. Body scans can cultivate a greater sense of resilience by helping you to develop a calm and centred response to stressors, enhancing self-awareness, and fostering a more adaptive mindset.

› The next is a chakra visualization that can also be a powerful tool to enhance resilience and cultivate a balanced and positive mindset. Chakras can be thought of as representing energy centres in the body that are associated with different aspects of physical, emotional and spiritual wellbeing. By using chakra visualizations, you can promote self-awareness, emotional regulation, and a sense of empowerment, all of which contribute to increased resilience. I've included an example of each in this book to help you get started with each practice.

› Finally we'll look at acceptance and a meditation on gratitude as powerful tools for empowerment and developing resilience.

› Remember that building resilience is an ongoing process. It's normal to face ups and downs, but by consistently practicing these strategies, you can strengthen your ability to navigate life's challenges with greater resilience, positivity and adaptability.

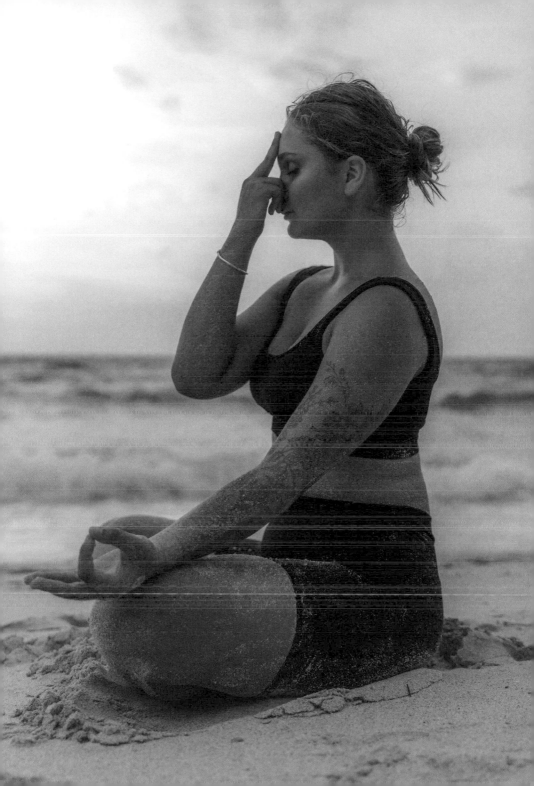

ACTIVITY: BODY SCAN & RESET

Take a moment to find a comfortable position, either sitting or lying down, where you can fully relax and let go of any tension in your body. Close your eyes gently, and bring your attention to your breath, allowing it to flow naturally. As you settle into a state of relaxation, we will begin a meditative body scan, focusing on each part of your body from the right toes, moving up through the body and back down to the left toes.

Begin by directing your attention to your right toes. Feel any sensations present in this area, whether warmth, tingling or a sense of stillness. Bring your awareness to the sole of your foot, noticing the points of contact with the ground or any sensations within. Gradually, shift your attention to the top of your foot, then to your ankle, feeling any feelings that arise.

Moving up, focus on your lower leg, noticing the muscles, bones, and any sensations you become aware of. Allow your awareness to gently move up to your knee, observing any sensations or subtle movements. Now, shift your attention to your upper leg, bringing awareness to your thigh and feeling any feelings present.

Continuing your journey through the body, focus on your pelvis and hips. Notice the weight of your body on the surface you're resting on. Be aware of any sensations, tensions, or areas of relaxation in this region. Moving up, direct your attention to your lower back, feeling the contact with the surface behind you and observing any sensations that arise.

Shifting your focus to your abdomen, notice the rise and fall of your breath in this area. Observe any feelings or sensations, allowing them to be. Now, bring your attention to your chest, feeling the gentle rhythm of your breath and any associated movements. Take a moment to appreciate the life-giving nature of each breath.

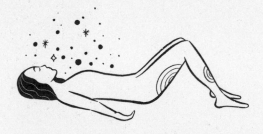

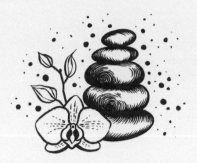

Moving up to your right hand, observe any sensations in your fingers, palm and back of your hand. Bring attention to your wrist, then gradually move up your forearm, feeling the muscles and bones. Shift your awareness to your elbow and upper arm, observing any sensations present.

Now, focus on your shoulder and collarbone, noticing any sensations. Shift your attention to your neck, feeling the muscles, bones, and any subtle movements associated with your breath. Finally, bring your awareness to your head, noticing any sensations in your face, jaw and temples. Observe any feelings on your scalp and the back of your head.

Now, slowly guide your awareness down the left side of your body, mirroring the path you took up the right side. Move through your neck, shoulder, arm, elbow, forearm and wrist. Observe any sensations in your left hand, fingers and palm. Continue down to your abdomen, lower back, hips and upper leg. Shift your focus to your knee, lower leg and left foot.

Take a moment to feel your entire body, from the top of your head to the tips of your toes. Observe any sensations present throughout your body without judgment or attachment. Allow yourself to momentarily rest in this calm awareness, breathing gently and deeply.

When you are ready, slowly open your eyes and reorient yourself to the space around you. Take this sense of calm and relaxation into the rest of your day, knowing you can return to this body scan practice whenever you need peace and self-awareness.

ACTIVITY: CHAKRA VISUALISATION

This is a meditative practice that involves focusing on and aligning the energy centres, or chakras, in the body. Each chakra is associated with specific physical, emotional and spiritual aspects, and by bringing awareness and balance to these energy centres, we can enhance our overall wellbeing and inner strength.

PREPARATION

Find a quiet and comfortable space where you won't be disturbed. Sit in a cross-legged position on the floor or on a chair with your spine straight and your hands resting on your knees or in a mudra of your choice (e.g. hands in Gyan Mudra with index finger and thumb touching).

Take a few deep breaths to relax and centre yourself. Close your eyes to turn your attention inward.

CHAKRA STRENGTHENING MEDITATION

Root Chakra (Muladhara): Bring your awareness to the base of your spine, the location of the root chakra. Visualise a deep earthy red light, gently suffusing the legs and lower half of your body. With each breath, imagine this red light expanding and becoming more vibrant, grounding you to the Earth and instilling a sense of safety and stability.

Sacral Chakra (Svadhishthana): Move your attention to the area just below your navel, where the sacral chakra is located. Visualise a burnt orange light, softly glowing at the base of your naval. As you breathe deeply, see the orange light growing brighter, stimulating creativity, and fostering a sense of emotional wellbeing.

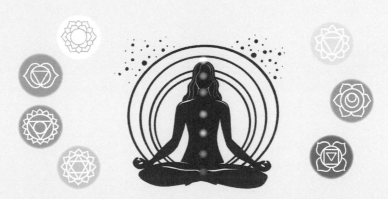

Solar Plexus Chakra (Manipura): Shift your focus to the area above your navel, where the solar plexus chakra resides. Envision a powerful yellow sun-bright light here. As you inhale and exhale, visualise the yellow light expanding and strengthening your sense of personal power, confidence and willpower.

Heart Chakra (Anahata): Bring your awareness to the centre of your chest, where the heart chakra is situated. Picture a beautiful, playful spring green light. With each breath, see the green light growing brighter, filling your heart with love, compassion, and forgiveness for yourself and others.

Throat Chakra (Vishuddha): Move your attention to your throat, the location of the throat chakra. Imagine a deep, ocean blue light. As you breathe deeply, visualise the blue light expanding and enhancing your ability to communicate clearly and authentically.

Third Eye Chakra (Ajna): Shift your focus to the centre of your forehead, between your eyebrows, where the third eye chakra is found. Visualise a pale violet light. With each breath, see this light growing brighter, opening your intuition and inner wisdom.

Crown Chakra (Sahasrara): Finally, bring your attention to the top of your head, the location of the crown chakra. Picture a radiant white light, connecting you to the universal consciousness. As you breathe deeply, envision this pure, brilliant light expanding, promoting spiritual connection and divine awareness.

INTEGRATION

Take a few moments to sit in stillness and allow the energy of the chakras to harmonise and integrate. Feel the flow of energy throughout your entire being, connecting all the chakras in a unified and balanced way.

When you are ready to end the practice, gently bring your awareness back to your surroundings. Open your eyes and take a moment to reflect on the experience.

Regularly practicing this meditation can enhance your sense of inner strength, emotional wellbeing and spiritual connection. As with any meditation, practice with an open heart, patience and self-compassion, allowing yourself to explore and deepen your relationship with your chakras and inner self.

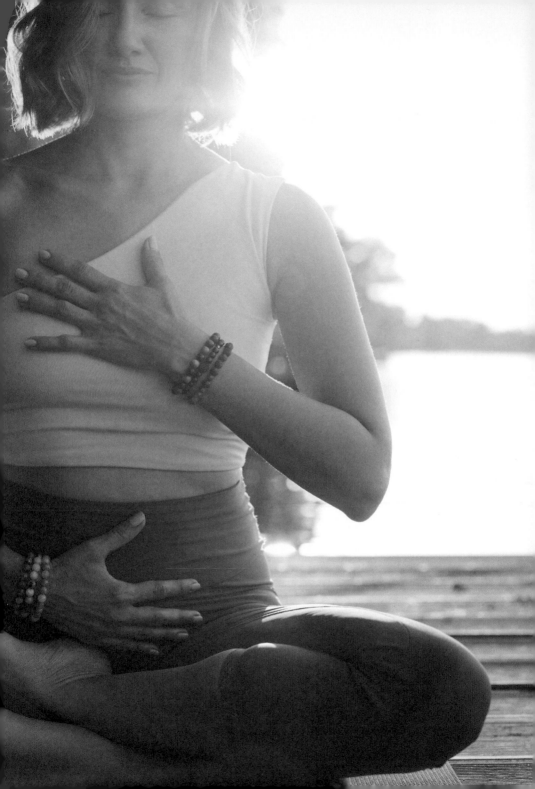

Moving Through Acceptance

The final lesson of this book, and one of the most important is accepting our bodies as they are.

A huge aspect of everything we've talked about concerns nurturing your mind and body where they are right now and not where you'd like them to be. This is something I have personally struggled with, and I need constant reminders to embrace the way I am – multiple sclerosis, thyroid issues and all. We must work with ourselves where we are and, in a world often driven by unrealistic standards of beauty and perfection, embracing our bodies and nurturing our inner selves becomes an act of empowerment and resilience. This journey encompasses understanding the interconnectedness of our physical, mental and emotional aspects, and finding balance and harmony amid the changes that life brings.

1. **Recognise the Natural Evolution:** Our bodies, minds and emotions are in constant flux due to the passage of time, experiences and external factors. Understanding that change is an inherent part of life can help us accept transitions gracefully. The body's aging process, its shifts in weight, and the ebb and flow of emotions are all natural phenomena that remind us of our shared human experience.

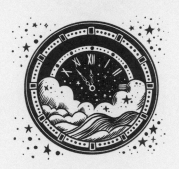

2. **Cultivate Self-Compassion:** Practice self-compassion by treating yourself with the same kindness and understanding you'd offer to a loved one. Acknowledge that imperfections are part of being human, and that your worth goes beyond physical appearance. Replace self-criticism with affirming and positive self-talk. I've included a final meditation on generating compassion to aid you with this practice.

3. **Embrace Mindfulness:** Mindfulness is a powerful tool to foster body acceptance. Engage in mindfulness practices that connect you to the present moment, allowing you to appreciate your body's sensations and functions without judgment. This practice can lead to greater body satisfaction and self-awareness.

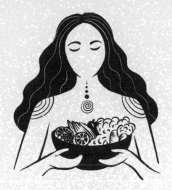

1. **Nourish Your Body with Intuitive Eating.** Practice intuitive eating by tuning into your body's hunger and fullness cues rather than adhering to restrictive diets. Trust your body's wisdom to guide your food choices and foster a healthy relationship with eating.

5. **Challenge Negative Beliefs:** Confront negative beliefs or societal standards that contribute to body dissatisfaction. Question where these beliefs originate and replace them with positive affirmations that emphasise your body's strengths, capabilities and uniqueness.

6. **Focus on Function over Appearance:** Shift your perspective from focusing solely on your body's appearance to appreciating its functionality and capabilities. Celebrate the ways your body allows you to move, engage in activities and experience life.

7. **Practice Gratitude:** Cultivate gratitude for your body's abilities and the experiences it enables. Shift your focus from what you perceive as flaws to what your body provides you every day.

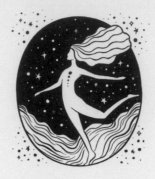

8. **Engage in Regular Physical Activity:** Engaging in regular physical activity not only contributes to physical wellbeing but also promotes mental and emotional health. Find forms of movement you enjoy, which can include walking, dancing, yoga, or any activity that makes you feel good.

9. **Seek Professional Support:** If grappling with body image concerns affects your mental and emotional wellbeing, consider seeking support from a therapist or counsellor. They can provide tools and strategies to navigate these challenges.

10. **Surround Yourself with Positivity:** Surround yourself with people who uplift and support you. Choose to engage with media and social content that promote body positivity, diversity and self-acceptance.

11. Focus on Inner Qualities: Shift the emphasis from external appearance to your inner qualities, talents and contributions. Remind yourself that your value extends far beyond physical attributes.

12. Embrace Emotional Expression: Allow yourself to experience a full range of emotions without judgment. Emotions are part of the human experience and acknowledging them contributes to overall wellbeing.

13. Connect with Like-minded Individuals: Connect with communities, groups or friends who share your values of body positivity and self-acceptance. Sharing experiences and perspectives can provide a sense of validation and support.

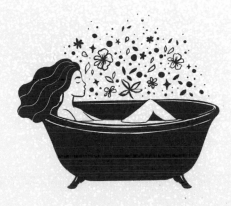

14. Practice Self-care Rituals: Engage in self-care activities that nurture your body, mind and emotions. These rituals can include meditation, journaling, taking baths, or spending time in nature.

15. Set Realistic Expectations: Recognise that perfection is unattainable and that comparing yourself to unrealistic standards can lead to dissatisfaction. Set realistic expectations for yourself and celebrate progress, no matter how small.

ACTIVITY: MEDITATION FOR COMPASSION

Compassion meditation, also known as loving-kindness meditation, is a practice that cultivates feelings of compassion, kindness and goodwill towards oneself and others. It is a powerful way to develop empathy, foster positive emotions, and enhance our connection with others. The practice typically involves repeating phrases or affirmations to evoke feelings of love and compassion.

PREPARATION

Find a quiet and comfortable place to sit in a cross-legged position on the floor or on a chair with your spine straight and your hands resting on your knees, or in a mudra of your choice.

Take a few deep breaths to relax and centre yourself. Close your eyes or soften your gaze to turn your attention inward.

COMPASSION MEDITATION

Start with self-compassion: begin by directing compassion towards yourself. Repeat the following phrases silently or aloud, focusing on their meaning and feeling the emotions they evoke:

May I be safe and protected.
May I be happy and peaceful.
May I be healthy and strong.
May I live with ease and joy.

EXPAND TO LOVED ONES

After cultivating self-compassion, extend your wishes of compassion to loved ones. Think of people you care about, such as family members, friends or mentors, and repeat the phrases for them:

May [name] be safe and protected.
May [name] be happy and peaceful.
May [name] be healthy and strong.
May [name] live with ease and joy.

EXTEND TO NEUTRAL PEOPLE

Next, think of people you have neutral feelings towards – acquaintances, colleagues or strangers. Extend your compassion to them as well:

May [name] be safe and protected.
May [name] be happy and peaceful.
May [name] be healthy and strong.
May [name] live with ease and joy.

INCLUDE DIFFICULT INDIVIDUALS

Now, challenge yourself to extend compassion to those with whom you have difficulties or conflicts. Practice generating compassion for them, acknowledging that they, too, deserve happiness and wellbeing:

May [name] be safe and protected.
May [name] be happy and peaceful.
May [name] be healthy and strong.
May [name] live with ease and joy.

EXPAND TO ALL BEINGS

Finally, extend your compassion universally to all living beings, near and far, human and non-human, without exception:

May all beings be safe and protected.
May all beings be happy and peaceful.
May all beings be healthy and strong.
May all beings live with ease and joy.

CONCLUSION

After completing the compassion meditation, sit in stillness for a few moments, experiencing the feelings of compassion and loving-kindness that you have cultivated.

When you are ready to end the practice, gently bring your awareness back to your surroundings. Open your eyes and take a moment to reflect on the experience.

Fostering your compassion

Practice compassion meditation regularly to develop and strengthen your sense of compassion and empathy.

Don't force feelings of compassion. If you encounter resistance or difficulty during the practice, be patient and gentle with yourself.

Customise the phrases to resonate with your personal beliefs and language.

As you progress in the practice, you can extend compassion to specific groups of people, such as those who are suffering or people in your community.

Compassion meditation is a profound practice that can transform our relationships with ourselves and others. It opens our hearts to the inherent goodness in all beings and fosters a sense of interconnectedness and unity. Embrace the power of compassion and let it ripple through your life, creating a positive impact on yourself and the world around you.

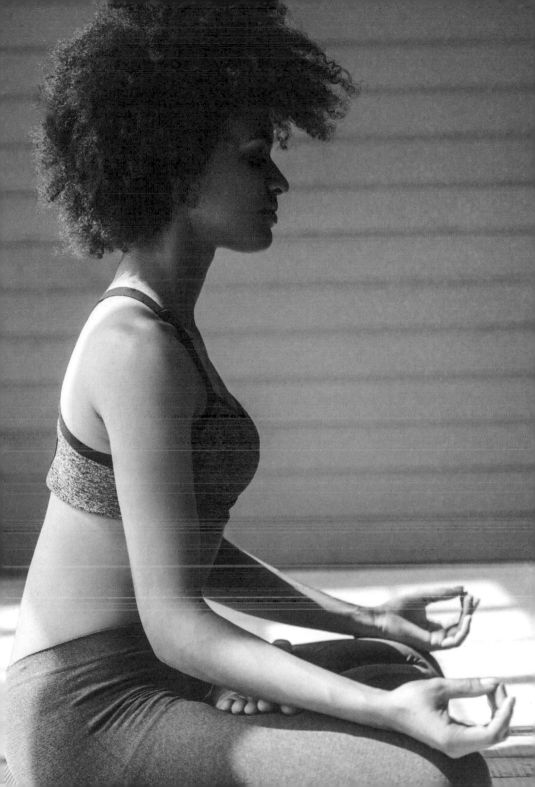

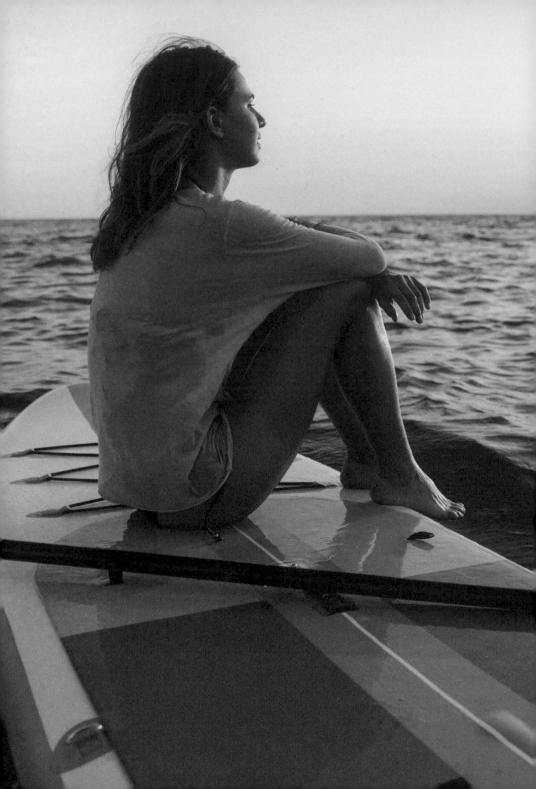

CONCLUSION

A Final Word on Movement

"Just as the ocean has waves or the sun has rays, so the mind's own radiance is its thoughts and emotions" Choje Lama Yeshe Losal Rinpoche, Lama of Tibetan Bhuddism, teacher and Abbot of the Kagyu Samye Ling Monastery

Accepting our bodies and navigating the changes that unfold over time is a journey of self-love, self-compassion and resilience. It involves embracing our bodies' natural evolution, cultivating self-awareness, and fostering a positive mindset. This journey is multifaceted, involving physical practices, mental shifts and emotional growth. Over time we can make the changes we need to truly utilise our energy and movement to heal and nourish our minds and bodies, working with them and never against them.

Somewhere in this book, I hope you have found your spark, your starting point, something that will help set you off on a quite different movement journey from the ones you have been on before. I hope you have found the gentler, self-caring side of practice that allows you to work with acceptance, compassion and trust for yourself.

It seems impossible to love ourselves compassionately one hundred per cent of the time and to hold that space to allow ourselves to grow, despite the fact we would do it for others. Partly, the reason behind writing this book was to serve as a reminder to do just that. To allow for 'failure', or even to enjoy failing and trying again. Something I say to my students when they fall out of balance or come to me with what they feel to be a setback, is that part of the practice is just simply re-setting. Let your preconceptions go and allow yourself to start again... and again, however many times you need to, as each time will bring you something slightly different.

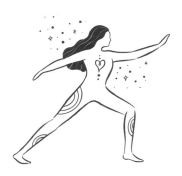

As a conclusion to this book, I have one final practice for you to try and adapt to your needs. A few years back, the 90 Days Hard challenge inundated my social media channels; it was a practice that promised to refine your entire being in just 90 days of hard work. The caveat was that if you failed a day, you had to restart the entire challenge, and in my view, the challenge was gruelling and somewhat impossible. You had to stick to a diet – it could be any diet, but you had to stick to it with no cheat days, no alcohol, and no sweets or candies. You also had to work out twice a day, for 45 minutes each time, and one of these sessions had to be outdoors. Finally, you had to read ten pages of non-fiction and drink excessive amounts of water. I commend those who managed to finish this challenge – however, I was not one of them. At the time, I devised an alternate challenge, a sort of '90 Days Soft' which worked on incorporating some of the elements that are now in this book.

INTRODUCING THE 90 DAY REFRAME

Understanding that I did not want to complete the 90 Days Hard was one of those moments of redefining what movement and what real joyful change would look like to me. Since then I have grown further and would like to share my updated version of a transformational practice: The 90 Day Reframe. For me, re-framing is about choosing to do one thing daily that works towards altering your long-held patterns. This could be in the form of how you notice the world on a walk, going for a jog or maybe a cold swim. It could be creating a nutritionally filling and healing meal that satisfies you and bolsters you against the elements. It could simply be clearing a space of the belongings you no longer need.

Over the 90 days your goal is to choose one thing per day and do it, then make a note in the planner on the following pages about the one thing you achieved. You could start with the practices from the book in any category—mind, body or breath—and see where it takes you, adding further ideas as you go. As you settle into the reframe you will hopefully become more intuitive about what brings you that sense of joy and freedom, what feels like it is bringing about a positive change for your physical, mental and spiritual wellbeing. If you find you miss a day – let it be ok, maybe note down what challenged you. Each day is a chance to begin again, and you can repeat the cycle as often as you'd like.

Finally, my last piece of advice is always to remember the playfulness and joy that movement can bring, to be out in nature as much as possible, and to reconnect with your ability to notice and be present. Enjoying movement through mind, body and breath is one of the most powerful tools we have in this world to engage authentically with the experiences around us and live our lives more compassionately.

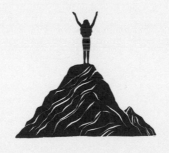

The 90 Day Reframe Planner

1	**2**	**3**	**4**	**5**
6	**7**	**8**	**9**	**10**
11	**12**	**13**	**14**	**15**
16	**17**	**18**	**19**	**20**
21	**22**	**23**	**24**	**25**
26	**27**	**28**	**29**	**30**

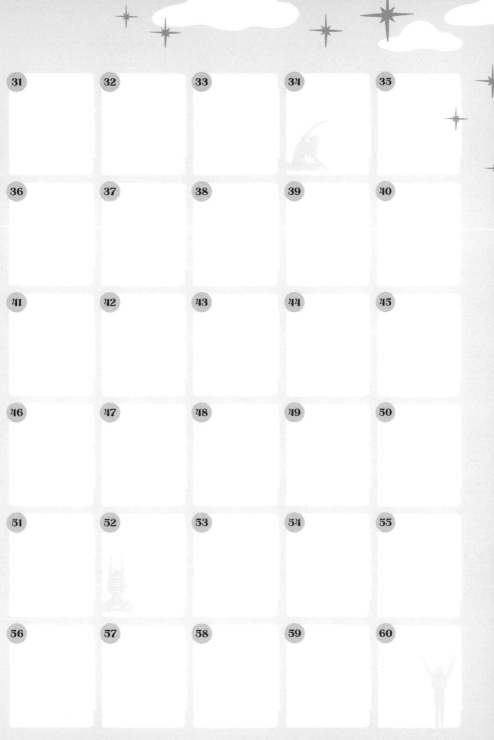

31	32	33	34	35
36	37	38	39	40
41	42	43	44	45
46	47	48	49	50
51	52	53	54	55
56	57	58	59	60

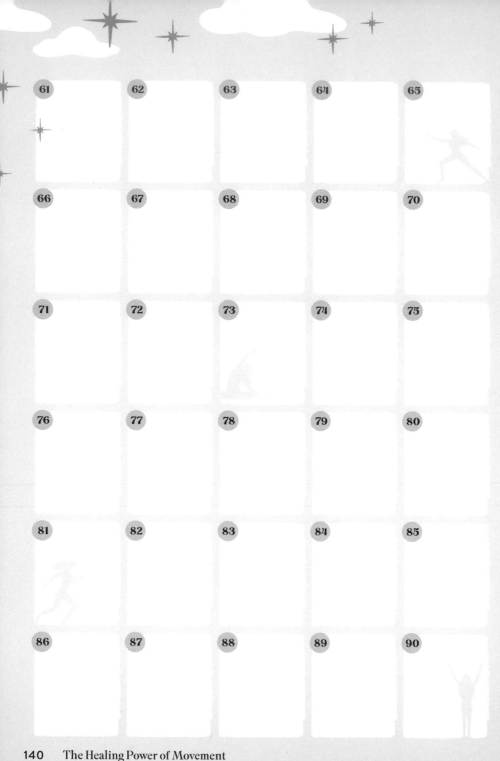

61	62	63	64	65
66	67	68	69	70
71	72	73	74	75
76	77	78	79	80
81	82	83	84	85
86	87	88	89	90

Further Reading

BOOKS

Benzie, Shane, The Lost Art of Running: A Journey to Rediscover the Forgotten Essence of Human Movement (Bloomsbury, London 2020)

Blackaby, Peter, *Intelligent Yoga* (Lotus Publishing, Chichester 2012)

Dweck, Carol, *Mindset: The New Psychology of Success* (Robinson, London 2006)

Hoban, Jonathan, Walk with Your Wolf: Unlock Your Intuition, Confidence and Power with Walking Therapy (Yellow Kite, London 2020)

Maté, Gabor, *When the Body Says No: Understanding the Stress-Disease Connection* (Vermilion, London 2003)

Nestor, James, *Breath: The New Science of a Lost Art* (Penguin Books, London 2020)

Rinpoche, Lama Yeshe Losal, *Living Dharma* (Dzalendara Publishing, Rokpa Trust, Scotland 2014)

Saraswati, Swami Satyananda, *Asana Pranayama Mudra Bandha* (Bihar School of Yoga, Munger 2008)

Shearer, Alistair, *The Yoga Sutras of Patanjali* (Element, London 2010)

Stirk, John, *The Original Body: Primal Movement for Yoga Teachers, Bodyworkers, and Movement Professionals* (Handspring Publishing, Edinburgh 2015)

The Yoga Sutras of Patanjali, trans. Georg Feuerstein (Shambhala, Boston 2014)

van der Kolk, Bessel, *The Body Keeps the Score: Brain, Mind, and Body in the Healing of Trauma* (Penguin Books, London 2015)

WEBSITES

Precision Nutrition: www.precisionnutrition.com

parkrun: www.parkrun.com

NHS Couch to 5k: www.nhs.uk/live-well/exercise/running-and-aerobic-exercises/get-running-with-couch-to-5k/

The Running Channel: www.runningchannel.com

The Outdoor Swimming Society: www.outdoorswimmingsociety.com

INDEX

A DAVID AND CHARLES BOOK
© David and Charles, Ltd 2024

David and Charles is an imprint of David and Charles, Ltd
Suite A, Tourism House, Pynes Hill, Exeter, EX2 5WS

Text © Hannah Glancy 2024
Layout and Illustration © David and Charles, Ltd 2024

First published in the UK and USA in 2024

Hannah Glancy has asserted her right to be identified as author of this work in accordance with the Copyright, Designs and Patents Act, 1988.

Names of manufacturers and product ranges are provided for the information of readers, with no intention to infringe copyright or trademarks.

A catalogue record for this book is available from the British Library.

ISBN-13: 9781446313176 paperback
ISBN-13: 9781446313350 EPUB

This book has been printed on paper from approved suppliers and made from pulp from sustainable sources.

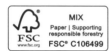

MIX
Paper | Supporting responsible forestry
FSC
www.fsc.org
FSC® C106499

Printed in Turkey by Omur for:
David and Charles, Ltd, Suite A, Tourism House, Pynes Hill, Exeter, EX2 5WS

10 9 8 7 6 5 4 3 2 1

Publishing Director: Ame Verso
Senior Commissioning Editor: Lizzie Kaye
Managing Editor: Jeni Chown
Editor: Jessica Cropper
Project Editor: Jane Trollope
Head of Design: Anna Wade
Design and Illustration: Prudence Rogers
Pre-press Designer: Susan Reansbury
Production Manager: Beverley Richardson

David and Charles publishes high-quality books on a wide range of subjects.
For more information visit www.davidandcharles.com.

Follow us on Instagram by searching for @dandcbooks_wellbeing.

Layout of the digital edition of this book may vary depending on reader hardware and display settings.